DOES YOUR NOSE RUN CONTINUOUSLY FROM THE MOMENT THE FIRST BUDS APPEAR ON THE TREES?

DO YOU BREAK OUT IN HIVES AND START TO ITCH WHENEVER YOU EAT CERTAIN FOODS?

DO YOU FIND YOURSELF WHEEZING AFTER BRIEF PERIODS OF EXERCISE?

DO YOUR EYES FREQUENTLY FEEL ITCHY AND WATERY?

If you have experienced any or all of these reactions, you are probably one of the more than 35 million Americans who suffer from allergies or asthma. You may have been born with certain allergies; you may develop them later in life; you may even develop immunity to one irritant only to find yourself suddenly sensitized to another. Pollens, foods, mold spores, insects, animals, and medications are just a few of the things that may provoke allergic reactions. But now you can find out everything you need to know about symptoms, causes, treatments, and where to go for help in

THE ALLERGY ENCYCLOPEDIA

RAYMOND G. SLAVIN, M.D. is President of the American Academy of Allergy and Immunology, former chairman of the Medical Advisory Council of the Asthma & Allergy Foundation of America and Director of the Allergy and Immunology section of the Medical School of the St. Louis University Medical Center.

CRAIG T. NORBACK, who edited this volume in conjunction with The Asthma & Allergy Foundation of America, has previously edited *The New American Guide to Athletics, Sports, & Recreation, The Complete Book of American Surveys,* and *The Signet Book of World Winners.*

THE
ALLERGY
ENCYCLOPEDIA

EDITED BY

THE ASTHMA &
ALLERGY FOUNDATION OF AMERICA
AND CRAIG T. NORBACK

Consulting Editor
Raymond G. Slavin, M.D.

A PLUME BOOK

NEW AMERICAN LIBRARY

NEW YORK AND SCARBOROUGH, ONTARIO

MOSBY MEDICAL LIBRARY

NAL BOOKS ARE AVILABLE AT QUANTITY DISCOUNTS
WHEN USED TO PROMOTE PRODUCTS OR SERVICES. FOR
INFORMATION PLEASE WRITE TO PREMIUM MARKETING DIVISION
NEW AMERICAN LIBRARY, 1633 BROADWAY,
NEW YORK, NEW YORK 10019.

SIGNET, SIGNET CLASSIC, MENTOR, PLUME, MERIDIAN
and NAL BOOKS are published *in the United States* by
New American Library,
1633 Broadway, New York, New York 10019,
in Canada by The New American Library of Canada Limited,
81 Mack Avenue, Scarborough, Ontario M1L 1M8.

Mosby Books are published by
The Mosby Press, The C. V. Mosby Company,
11830 Westline Industrial Drive, St. Louis, Missouri 63141

First Printing, August, 1981

First Mosby Medical Library Printing, May, 1982

8 9 10 11 12 13 14

PRINTED IN THE UNITED STATES OF AMERICA

Contents

v

Contributors

RAYMOND G. SLAVIN, M.D., is President of the American Academy of Allergy and Immunology and former Chairman of the Medical Advisory Council of the Asthma & Allergy Foundation of America. He is a professor of internal medicine and microbiology at the St. Louis University School of Medicine.

JOHN E. SALVAGGIO, M.D., is Henderson Professor of Medicine at Tulane University School of Medicine. He has published and lectured extensively on immunology and related medical subjects.

HAROLD S. NOVEY, M.D., is clinical professor of medicine at the University of California, Irvine, and Chief of the Division of Allergy-Immunology, Department of Medicine, University of California, Irvine, Medical Center.

THOMAS M. GOLBERT, M.D., is assistant clinical professor of medicine at the University of Colorado School of Medicine. He has a private practice in allergy and clinical immunology.

WILLIAM R. SOLOMON, M.D., is a professor of internal medicine at the University of Michigan Medical School.

MANUEL LOPEZ, M.D., is assistant clinical professor of medicine at Tulane University Medical School and director of the Immunology Diagnosis Laboratory in Pensacola, Florida.

DAVID A. LEVY, M.D., is professor of biochemistry and medicine at The Johns Hopkins University. He has lectured and published on the mechanism of immediate hypersensitivity.

GAIL G. SHAPIRO, M.D., is clinical associate professor of pediatrics at the University of Washington, Seattle, and a frequent writer on allergy-related subjects.

SHELDON L. SPECTOR, M.D., is head of the section in allergy of the National Jewish Hospital and Research Center, Denver, Colorado, and associate professor of medicine at the University of Colorado Medical Center.

Foreword

This book is dedicated to the thirty-five million Americans (and their families) who suffer from allergies. Allergies are the most common form of chronic disease in the United States. Nine million Americans suffer from asthma, almost fifteen million have hay fever, and another twelve million have such allergic diseases as eczema, hives, angioedema, food and drug sensitivity, and insect sting hypersensitivity. All told, 17 percent of Americans are allergic to some degree. Clearly, we are dealing with a condition with enormous importance to public health.

The impact of these diseases is considerable. In some cases, the financial burden may overwhelm families. The total cost of allergic diseases to American society as a whole has been estimated at more than $1 billion. The direct cost—including physician services, hospital care, and medication—is $850 million; the indirect cost, such as days lost from work, runs into the hundreds of millions of dollars.

Other, more subtle, costs are involved, which have to do with the quality of life for Americans. Activity is often restricted, work may have to be limited to certain areas, and both physical and emotional growth may be retarded. The special demands of an allergic person can place a substantial strain on his or her family. Vacations must be restricted, family income diverted, and activity around the home limited—all of which can affect the nonallergic members of a family almost as much as the allergic one. Is it any wonder, then, that the divorce rate among allergic families is significantly higher than it is among families without allergic members?

The Allergy Encyclopedia is designed to provide the allergy sufferer, as well as friends and families, with an overall view of this common, complex group of diseases. With knowledge comes understanding. Our hope is that the distinguished doctors represented in this encyclopedia have accomplished their mission to dispel myths and provide readers with up-to-date, readable, and medically accurate information.

To understand and control allergic diseases, we must first understand the immune system. Dr. Levy sets the stage with a clear exposition of immunology—the basic science of allergy. Dr. Solomon discusses regional factors in allergy and provides the reader with an overview of the various inhalants around the country that may be responsible for allergic diseases. A guide to allergies by doctors Lopez and Salvaggio, in glossary form, defines the terms most often encountered. Drugs commonly used to treat allergies are covered by Dr. Golbert, and the most serious of the allergic diseases—namely, allergic emergencies—are covered by Dr. Novey. Dr. Shapiro describes research in immunology and discusses the various approaches to the treatment of allergies, showing graphically how scientists in the laboratory are attempting to provide the basic information that could lead to clinical advances in diagnosis and treatment. A separate chapter is devoted to questions frequently asked about allergic diseases. Finally, a special effort has been made in this book to provide information of practical use to the reader. Included are a listing of allergy associations, summer camps, residential centers, and hospitals, as well as diets and cooking hints and a suggested reading list.

This Foreword would not be complete without mention of The Asthma & Allergy Foundation of America, the major national voluntary health organization concerned with these widespread immunologic diseases. A nonprofit organization formed over thirty years ago, AAFA's goal is the control and cure of asthma and allergic disease through stimulating growth in the science of immunology; training future leaders in allergy and immunology; aiding the continuing medical education of physicians and other health care providers; and, most important, creating more—and more informed—choices for over 35 million sufferers, their families, and friends. AAFA supports the scientific studies of brilliant physician-scientists in immunology through financial awards, aids specialized clinical training in immunology with annual fellowships, helps sponsor continuing medical education programs at leading medical institutions, works at the grassroots to support and educate patients and families, and conducts local and national drives to raise public concern and financial support for healthier Americans with asthma and allergic diseases. AAFA's Medical-Scientific Council, its source of current scientific and professional knowledge, is a service of the American Academy of Allergy and Immunology. The address of the Headquarters Office of AAFA, which strongly deserves our support, is: 1302 18th Street NW, Suite 303, Washington, D.C. 20036. (A list of AAFA chapters is found on pages 242-243.)

Acknowledgments

The editors wish to thank the following persons and organizations for their contributions to the present volume: The Asthma & Allergy Foundation of America; National Institute of Allergy and Infectious Diseases; M. Susan Daglish, Allergy Information Association; American Academy of Allergy and Immunology; Carol Rudoff, American Allergy Association; *Annals of Allergy*; W. B. Saunders Company; Syracuse University Press; Abbott Laboratories; Fran Gentile; Bobbi Angell; Phil Jones; Hollister-Stier Laboratories.

We wish to make a special acknowledgment to the late Dr. Francis Cabot Lowell, who at the time of his death was consulting editor of this volume. Long associated with the allergy unit of Massachusetts General Hospital, Boston, and with Harvard Medical School, Dr. Lowell had begun to bring his lifetime of expertise to this book, as he did to his work generally. He will be missed.

THE
ALLERGY
ENCYCLOPEDIA

CHAPTER 1

Questions Frequently Asked about Allergies

Allergic Diseases

Just what is an allergy?
An allergy is an abnormal reaction to an ordinarily harmless substance or substances. These substances, called allergens, may be inhaled, swallowed, injected, or contacted by the skin.

What are some common allergens?
There are many possible allergens. For example: pollen, mold, and house dust; animal dander (skin shed by dogs, cats, horses, rabbits, and so on); feathers (as in old-fashioned pillows); kapok, wool, dyes, and industrial chemicals; foods and medicines; and insect stings.

What does an allergen do in the body?
When an allergen is absorbed into the bloodstream, it stimulates certain small white blood cells called lymphocytes to produce special substances known as allergic antibodies. These antibodies react with the allergen and produce allergic inflammation and irritation in particularly sensitive areas of the body, such as the nose, eyes, lungs, or digestive system. This sensitivity is not present at first contact with the allergen; instead, it may develop after repeated exposure. For example, a new cat may not cause allergy until it has been living in a house for many months. Eventually, a susceptible person becomes sensitized and develops a stuffy nose and sneezing or wheezing on further contact with the cat.

What are some allergic diseases?
Allergic diseases or reactions can involve any part of the body. The parts, or systems, most frequently involved are the respiratory system, where an allergic reaction may take the form of hay fever (allergic rhinitis) and asthma, and the skin, where a reaction can take the form of allergic dermatitis or atopic eczema, contact dermatitis (for

example, poison ivy), or hives (urticaria). An allergic disease may
also be a factor in numerous other diseases.

Hay fever is caused by allergy to the pollen of trees, grasses, weeds,
or molds, or any combination of these. Depending on the section of
the United States (unless otherwise indicated, this means the conti-
nental United States) and the pollinating periods, it may occur in the
spring, summer, or fall, and it may last until the first frost. The hay
fever sufferer has spells of sneezing, itching, weeping eyes, running
nose, and a burning sensation in the palate and throat.

Allergic rhinitis is a general term that applies to anyone with nasal
congestion, sneezing, and a running nose—all caused by allergies.
This may be a seasonal problem, as with hay fever, or it may be a
year-round problem caused by other allergens such as house dust,
animal dander, and perhaps some foods. Because allergic rhinitis is
frequently confused with sinusitis, patients with constant nasal symptoms should be evaluated for allergies.

Asthma is a condition characterized by coughing, wheezing, and
difficulty breathing. It is frequently, but not invariably, associated with
a family history of allergy. Any of the previously mentioned allergens
can precipitate asthma attacks. Infections of the sinuses or the bronchial tubes may also be an important factor. Asthma patients are
adversely affected by such "nonspecific" factors as air pollutants,
cigarette smoke, and fumes. Their own emotions sometimes come into
play. Asthma may begin at any age. If neglected, it tends to recur and
become chronic.

Allergic dermatitis, or *eczema*, is a noncontagious, itchy rash that
often occurs in the creases of the arms, legs, and neck, although it
sometimes covers the entire body. The condition is frequently associated with allergies, and substances to which a person is sensitive can
aggravate it. Foods are known to cause allergic dermatitis. A family
history of allergy is thought to be a factor in its occurrence.

Contact dermatitis is a rash caused by direct skin contact with any
of a variety of substances—animal, plant, chemical, or mineral. The
most common cause is poison ivy.

Urticaria, or *hives*, is an outbreak on the skin of itchy welts of varying size. When the welts are large and invade deeper tissues, they are
called angioedema. They may develop on the face, lips, tongue,
throat, eyes, ears, or even internally. Allergies to food or drugs (especially penicillin) are well-known causes, but hives may also result
from an underlying disease, or the disease may occur after emotional
stress. Sometimes the exact cause cannot be determined.

Is a particular age group prone to allergy?
No. Allergy may develop in people of any age. Even infants some-

times exhibit symptoms of allergy, and some people experience their first attacks of allergy in middle age or later. Nevertheless, children are more likely to develop allergies than are people later in life.

Do many people suffer from allergic diseases?
Statistics compiled by the National Institute of Allergy and Infectious Diseases show that thirty-five million people suffer from allergy and that nine million of this group have asthma.

Allergy Diagnosis, Treatment, and Prevention

Is early diagnosis important?
Yes. Asthma in childhood, if neglected, can lead to serious, disabling lung disease in adult life. Unfortunately, the notion that an asthmatic child will outgrow the condition is not true. Asthma that is not diagnosed early and treated effectively can lead to physical retardation and personality problems that will handicap the child throughout life. Early diagnosis and treatment, not only in children but in adults as well, can prevent serious complications later on.

How do I find out what caused my allergy?
Your doctor, in addition to taking a thorough history of your illness, may make a study of your home and work environment, your diet, and your living habits. The doctor will also give you a physical examination and run some laboratory tests. Using extracts of common allergens, the doctor may perform various skin tests to ascertain allergies to specific allergens. After reviewing the family history, giving an examination, and running skin tests, the physician will be able to determine whether you have an allergy or allergies and, if so, what allergens are involved. This requires planning, skill, and patience. An accurate diagnosis cannot be obtained simply by performing allergy tests alone, as is done in some testing laboratories.

What can I—or anyone—do about an allergic disease?
Whenever allergens in a patient's environment can be isolated, they should. This is fairly easy when a feather pillow or dust-catching furniture is the problem. When a person is sensitive to a cat, dog, or bird, however, removing the allergen source may not be easy because of an emotional attachment. It can be done, though, by using patience and compassion and by explaining the risk of keeping the pet. If foods are the cause of the difficulty, they must be eliminated from the diet.
The timing and proper use of medications are important in treat-

ing allergic disease. A medical doctor must prescribe the medications and their dosages. Numerous medications are now available that are helpful both in preventing symptoms and in providing relief from them. They may be all that is needed in cases of mild allergy. If symptoms persist despite the proper use of medications and the removal of allergens from the environment, immunizing injections may be necessary to control the disease.

Is good general health important?
Yes. The best way to achieve and maintain good health is with a balanced diet and a well-rounded program of exercise, recreation, and rest. Smoking is extremely harmful and, in the case of the allergy sufferer, must be avoided. Although these measures will not cure an allergy, they do contribute to better resistance.

People say allergy is psychosomatic. Is this true?
It is true that such emotions as anxiety, fear, anger, and strong excitement can precipitate allergic attacks or make an existing condition suddenly worse. This is not to say, however, that these emotions are the physical basis of the allergy—which is real and of primary importance to people with allergies. Few patients need psychological help, but a child with severe asthma may cause serious disturbance in family life. In such cases, counselling for other members of the patient's family is of great benefit as an auxiliary to medical treatment. In general, the allergic patient is better off in an atmosphere of calm and confidence. Parents of asthmatic children should, as much as possible, maintain an attitude of calm and reassurance. The allergic child should be encouraged to be self-reliant and to take part in all activities to the extent possible.

Would a change of climate benefit me?
A hay fever victim may find relief by moving to an area where the offending allergen, pollen, or mold is not present. Some asthmatics, especially those whose asthma is caused by infection or complicated by it, may benefit from a warm, dry climate. Before a change of climate is recommended, however, the climate sought should be studied thoroughly and comprehensively. The change itself is not as important as proper treatment and, where possible, removal of the allergen. In most cases, moving to another area does not cause the allergy problem to improve. When a move is not practical—for economic, professional, or other reasons—air-conditioning and such other home-filtration devices as electronic air cleaners may be helpful. Working against air pollution through citizen clean air groups is another, al-

beit more long-range, way to reduce airborne allergens in one's own community.

Can allergic disease be prevented?

Generally, people who are aware of their problems can avoid offending allergens by not walking or driving in the country during the pollen season; by avoiding drafts and exposure to cold, damp air; by keeping away from house dust; by trying not to breathe the fumes of paint, insecticides, or products containing irritants; by not using or coming in contact with aerosols, cosmetics, dyes, or strong cleansers. Allergic people should strive to keep in good physical condition and to avoid emotional tension and fatigue. When they occur, respiratory infections should be taken seriously and treated early. It is especially important that parents watch children for allergic tendencies.

Foods are a common cause of allergy in infancy. Breast milk is preferable to cow's milk in potentially allergic children. Eggs, raw vegetables, and fruits should be added to the diet one at a time, and the child's reaction should be monitored. Bedrooms and play areas should be as dust-free as possible, and dogs and cats should be avoided.

Is it dangerous to ignore an allergy?

In some cases, yes. Severe hay fever, if left untreated, can lead to nasal polyps and sinusitis. Patients with allergic rhinitis who also have nasal polyps should undergo allergic evaluation and therapy to help prevent further growth of the polyps. Allergic dermatitis, or eczema, that is not treated early can spread and occasionally be complicated by secondary infection. The patient who originally has only occasional periods of asthma may develop a chronic condition. If the allergies are detected early, however, and appropriate treatment is begun, the condition may improve or at least be controlled.

Can an allergy be fatal?

Allergic disorders are seldom fatal, though it is estimated that about five thousand people in the United States die each year from asthma. There are approximately forty deaths each year from allergic reactions to insect stings. Reactions from some drugs, and from certain foods such as nuts and seafoods, have occasionally proved fatal. Asthmatic patients are at additional risk when undergoing surgery that involves anesthesia.

Can I ever be cured of my allergy?

In many patients, the tendency to allergy is inherited. Because this predisposition to allergy may remain for life, it is not possible to speak of a "cure." This does not mean, though, that allergic conditions cannot be controlled to the point where the patient is symptom-free and can lead a virtually normal life. Early investigation of allergies, removal of offending allergens, timely and correct use of new drugs for symptomatic relief of allergic diseases, and improvements in immunization have led to a high success rate in the treatment of allergic diseases. Many more allergy sufferers can benefit from the dissemination of information about allergies and their treatment and by providing better medical facilities.

I am twenty-three and would like to have a child. I hesitate to do so, however, because of my long history of allergies and asthma. I take cromolyn sodium capsules. My doctor advises me to discontinue the drug while I am pregnant, but my allergist said I could continue the drug. What should I do?

According to the instructions accompanying cromolyn sodium, its dosage and frequency of use during pregnancy have not been established, because no controlled, clinical trials have been performed among pregnant users. The drug has few known side effects, however, in general use, and has been found useful in some cases of asthma. Although most allergists continue to prescribe cromolyn sodium for pregnant women, the decision ultimately is the patient's. At any rate, use of the drug—or of any medication—during the first trimester should be kept to the smallest dosage compatible with the control of symptoms. The pregnant woman should rely on the advice of her allergist, who is likely to be more knowledgeable about asthma medication than the obstetrician.

I am pregnant and am currently taking weekly allergy shots for grass and dust. My child is allergic to milk and soybean formulas. Is it possible to prevent allergies in my unborn child?

There is no certain way to prevent the development of allergies in the children of allergic parents, but here are some suggestions:

1. Breastfeed the baby. When the child is weaned, use evaporated milk rather than whole cow's milk. If soybean milk formula does not cause diarrhea, that may be used.

2. When cereals are added to the diet, use single ones rather than mixtures. That way, causative agents can be identified more readily if trouble develops.

3. Feed the baby no eggs, chocolate, or orange juice during the first year. Vitamin drops may be substituted for orange juice.

4. Do not let wool come in contact with the baby's skin.

5. Do not allow pets in the house.

6. Use water- and dust-proof covers on the child's mattress, as well as acrylon pillows, instead of those made with feathers. This rule also applies to stuffed animals; choose toys of acrylon or foam rubber.

I have heard of a drug called Intal that is supposed to help asthma patients. What is this drug, and would it be safe for a diabetic to use?

Intal is the trade name for sodium cromolyn, a powder that is inhaled into the lungs. It can be useful both in preventing asthma and as a medication. Intal, however, contains a small amount (20 milligrams per capsule) of lactose sugar, something your physician, if aware of your condition, will take into consideration. Other than this, there should be no problem in using this medication.

Is it possible for an asthmatic to tolerate cigarette smoke?

Because tobacco smoke is noxious (that is, it consists of such gases as carbon monoxide and particulates), an asthma patient is apt to experience difficulty when exposed to it. Thus tobacco smoke should be avoided as much as possible.

My seventeen-year-old-daughter is a chronic asthmatic and has been so since infancy. She is often absent from school because of her allergy, and the pressures of school build up, which greatly aggravates her condition. Is there anything I can do?

A note from your physician to the principal (or, in rare cases, the school board) should help. Perhaps special arrangements can be made for tutoring at home. Since stress, as you suggest, aggravates your daughter's condition, everything possible should be done to remove pressures from her daily life.

Our son, who is three-and-a-half, suffers from bronchial asthma. Would lowering the humidity in our house make it easier for him to breathe?

Asthmatic patients generally do better in an atmosphere of constant humidity. A low-humidity environment is usually best. Even in the best-controlled patients, however, many things can precipitate an asthma attack, for example, cold air, noxious fumes, emotional stress, and infections.

I am an asthmatic. I have various allergies to such substances as dust, pollen, and some foods. Recently I developed a sensitivity to synthetic fabrics. Is there anything I can do about this new allergy?

The chemical coating of many artificial fibers, rather than the fibers themselves, can provoke allergic reactions. Most of these reactions are caused by direct contact, which produces a form of contact dermatitis. The best approach is to wash new clothes repeatedly before wearing them, to leach out the allergenic coating.

Food Allergy

I have had digestive upsets from milk, citric and ascorbic acids, aspirin, coffee, and tea. The doctor told me to eliminate from my diet all foods that disagree with me. Is he right?

It is true that the best treatment for a food allergy is simply to avoid eating the food. Other than this, about all that can be done is to find substitutes for the offending substances. Most people who are allergic consider themselves fortunate that they have been able to identify the foods that caused the reactions.

My two-year-old daughter is allergic to milk. Is there any chance that she will outgrow this allergy?

Sensitivity to milk and other foods is not uncommon in children, and the sensitivity does tend to be outgrown. Although there is a good chance that a sensitivity will diminish in time, physicians have no way of knowing for sure whether a sensitivity will persist.

When I weaned my son from breast milk and began feeding him cow's milk, he began to have digestive problems. I stopped the cow's milk, but now I am worrying about replacing the vitamins and minerals he would normally get from that milk. What should I do?

A number of substitutes for cow's milk are available, including meat-base and soy-milk formulas. Your physician should be able to prescribe one. If the child shows signs of other allergies, an allergist can advise you on the necessary medication and treatment.

My doctor told me I have an egg allergy. How can I find out what foods contain eggs, so that I can avoid eating them? Also, is it better to seek advice on this subject from an allergist or from a doctor who is nutrition-oriented?

For best results, it is helpful to eliminate those foods you suspect are aggravating your allergy. Obtain a diet from your physician and make it a habit to read the labels of foods you buy. If you are not sure of a food's ingredients, don't eat the food. Experience has shown that an allergist is more attuned to allergy-related food problems than is a nutrition-oriented physician.

My ten-month-old son seems to have stomach cramps and gas any time he is given food containing soybean. Is this an unusual problem?

Sensitivity to soybean is an increasingly apparent problem. Most children outgrow this sensitivity. While they remain sensitive, though, soybean should be avoided in any form. Soybean-containing foods can be avoided by reading labels.

Do you have any information on the swelling of salivary glands caused by allergies? When I eat certain foods, my glands begin to swell, and my saliva stops.

Swelling of the salivary glands may be a manifestation of an allergic reaction to a food. Once you have identified the food or foods responsible for this reaction, the only recourse is to avoid them. Other causes of salivary-gland swelling—for example, stenosis, or narrowing, of the salivary duct and infection—should be ruled out. Your doctor will help determine the exact cause.

Allergies Related to the Upper Respiratory System

I have perennial rhinitis and chronic sinusitis. It seems that whenever there is a change in the weather, I have trouble keeping my balance. Can the weather affect or aggravate my condition?

Evidence is increasing that various weather phenomena, including changes in barometric pressure, have a significant effect on human health. With regard to your particular problem, it is best to seek a physician's advice and help in administering nasal decongestants when the weather changes, to minimize the effects of the changes.

I am troubled by an excess amount of postnasal drip, which clogs my vocal chords and makes me hoarse. I have had polyps removed several times in the past. Is there anything that can be done to alleviate the problem?

Both researchers and doctors believe that one of the causes of nasal polyposis is a chronic allergic state. This condition, coupled with postnasal drip, could well be responsible for your hoarseness. A complete allergic survey should be made, followed by therapy.

I have lost my sense of smell. Could this be caused by an allergy? Can it be treated?

Allergy could indeed be causing you to lose your sense of smell. If all other possible causes have been eliminated, an allergic survey is needed. This survey, which may include skin tests, may be able to identify the external substances to which you are allergic. It is possible that a specific treatment will be prescribed, based on the information turned up by the survey.

Animal-Related Allergies

We had a dog for two years before our son became asthmatic. How could the dog be the cause if the asthma took so long to develop?
No one is allergic to a substance the first time it is encountered; a period of sensitization precedes the onset of the allergy. Two years is a typical period, though some allergies appear sooner and some later.

Is it safe to have a pet that does not shed?
The allergen from dogs or cats that causes an allergic reaction is not present in the hair of the animal, but rather in the dander, or flakes of the animal's skin.

Is it all right to have a pet if it is outside most of the time?
It takes only a few minutes for sufficient dander to accumulate on carpets and furniture. This is why allergic individuals have problems even when a pet is kept in the basement. When the pet is removed from the house, and after thorough cleaning, it may take up to four weeks for the dander to dissipate.

Can't I just receive shots for my allergy to dogs?
Allergy injections for sensitivity to animal dander are not advisable except in unusual circumstances. One circumstance is the blind person who becomes allergic to a seeing-eye dog; another is the small-animal veterinarian who becomes allergic to house pets. The most effective course of action is to remove the pet from the environment.

I have two children who are allergic to pollen and mold. They have never had problems around animals. Is it safe to give them a dog or a cat?
Allergic children are predisposed to allergies to new substances. A casual encounter, such as visiting friends who have a pet, may not be enough to sensitize a child; but continued, massive exposure to an animal will often do so. Unfortunately, this sensitization frequently takes one to two years, which means that the new allergy becomes evident just as the pet becomes an integral part of the family, and just when separation is the most traumatic. The best advice is simply not

to have a dog, cat, or other fur-bearing animal in a home where a family member is allergic. Some pets that are safe for allergic families are tropical fish, turtles, chameleons, iguanas, and snakes.

Allergies to Single or Multiple Environmental Factors

I have an allergy to cosmetics, specifically to face makeup, lipstick, and powder. Is there anything that can be done?

Allergies to cosmetics are extremely common. The best approach is to use only those that are *truly* hypoallergenic, that is, cosmetics that do not contain common allergens. Such companies as AR-EX, Alcon (Allercreme), Almay, and Clinique market cosmetics that are claimed to be nonallergenic.

My daughter is allergic to a chemical called mercaptobenzothiazole, used in the shoe-manufacturing process. What can be done about this allergy?

Mercaptobenzothiazole, widely used in manufacturing shoes, is used in processing all leather. For a complete cure, contact with leather should be avoided. When this isn't possible, the condition can be alleviated by keeping the feet as dry as possible, using a powder such as Zea-sorb, or by applying creams and lotions to heal active lesions and using nonmedicated creams or ointments to keep the skin soft. A dermatologist or an allergist can advise you further.

I am sensitive to perfume and smoke. When I am exposed to either or both, I have difficulty breathing, and blisters develop in my mouth, throat, and lungs. Is there anything I can do?

Aside from the recognized fact that perfume and smoke are irritants, little is known about what causes respiratory difficulties or the blisters. Until researchers discover an effective means of desensitizing a patient against the effect of such agents, the best advice is to stay away from them.

My husband seems to be allergic to dust, atmospheric molds, ragweed, grass, and trees. At night the back of his throat swells up, and he finds it hard to breathe. What can we do about it?

The type of reaction you describe—the "swelling" is of the uvula, flesh that hangs in the back of the throat—may well be caused by an allergy. The inhalants you mention, however, are less likely causes of the problem than are foods or medications. To determine the causes precisely, you should seek the advice of an allergist. Then appropriate remedies can be prescribed.

My nine-year-old son is allergic to numerous pollens, molds, and foods, for which he takes weekly injections. He is also hyperactive. Is there any relationship between his allergies and the hyperactivity?
The relationship between allergies and hyperactivity, or hyperkinesis, remains to be proved. Although controlled studies are not available, most allergists believe that no relationship exists.

I suffer from reactions to ragweed and dust and have been taking shots for the last four years, with no sign of improvement. Would I be better off taking dust from my own house to an allergist? Have there been any new developments in the allergy field? Are there any antihistamines that would be effective?
For certain patients, an extract of dust from your house would be more useful in treatment than the commercially produced extracts formulated to be like those that originate in most households. Usually, however, there must be a peculiar condition in your home for the dust to differ.

There are no new, significant developments in the treatment of allergic rhinitis that your doctor would not be likely to know about, considering today's communications and the dissemination of scientific information. Ornade, CoPyronil, and Actifed, for example, are considered effective antihistamines and decongestants, but they cause drowsiness in some allergic people. You should discuss any questions about treatment with antihistamines with your physician.

I have a severe allergic reaction to dust. What is the proper treatment?
House-dust allergy is extremely common in the United States. Avoidance of dust, use of antihistamines, and desensitization injections are the usual therapeutic approaches, with avoidance the most important. Your allergist can advise you about how to avoid house dust.

I am allergic to mold and dust, and take shots for them. Injections affect my stomach, though, and make me nauseous. Is this normal?
A reaction of any sort after an allergy shot probably means that the dosage is too high and that it should be reduced. Seek the advice of the allergist who is providing you with the injections.

I used to wear contact lenses, but they began to irritate my eyes. Is this an allergic reaction?

It is indeed possible that you are experiencing an allergic reaction, perhaps because of the eye-drop solution used. The best way to determine this is to avoid such use for a period of time, say until your eyes clear up. If you then resume use of the product and your eyes again smart, burn, or swell, it is likely that you are allergic to the product.

I was tested for fifteen molds and found to be allergic to eleven of them. I am receiving desensitizing injections for only four of the molds. Why?

Allergy injections should include substances that are not only positive in skin testing but that are present in significant amounts in the outside air. Thus, in the case of mold sensitivity, the molds for which you are receiving injections are by far the most common in the outside air, whereas those for which you are not receiving injections are relatively unimportant in terms of their concentration in the air.

Do mites have any connection with house-dust allergy?

Yes. Many allergists believe that the household mite, a microscopic insect distantly related to the bedbug, is a primary factor in house-dust allergy.

CHAPTER 2

Allergies, Allergens, and Related Terms–A Guide
by Manuel Lopez, M.D.,
and John E. Salvaggio, M.D.

ACTH Adrenocorticotropic hormone, abbreviated ACTH, is a hormone that is produced by the pituitary gland. The hormone stimulates the production and release of corticosteroids (cortisone) by the adrenal gland.

Actinomycetes Actinomycetes are microorganisms that are closely related to bacteria. Abundant in soil, compost, fresh water, and other compounds, they are the source of antibiotics, vitamins, and enzymes. Actinomycetes are now known to be an important source of the antigens responsible for hypersensitivity pneumonitis, or allergic alveolitis, an immunological disease of the lungs. Some examples of hypersensitivity pneumonitis are farmer's lung, bagassosis, bird fancier's disease, and humidifier lung.

Adjuvant In medicine, adjuvant is a substance that, when added to an antigen, enhances the production of antibodies.

Adrenalin Adrenalin is a brand name for epinephrine, an extract of the hormone secreted by the adrenal gland; it is used as a treatment in some allergy emergencies.

Adrenergic Agonist *See* Bronchodilator.

Air Pollution Air pollution is the atmospheric accumulation of substances, usually artificial, to such an extent that the accumulation becomes harmful to humans, animals, and plants. The two main types of air pollution are industrial smog and photochemical smog.
Industrial smog is the most prevalent form of air pollution in large industrialized areas such as New York City and Chicago and their environs. Industrial smog is the result of the combustion of sulfur-containing fossil fuels, especially coal and some fuel oils.

14

Photochemical smog is the result of automobile and other exhaust emissions. It accumulates in areas such as Los Angeles and Denver, which are situated in basins and have a high density of motor vehicles and enough sunlight for a photochemical reaction to take place.

Clearly, air pollution aggravates respiratory problems. Because people with asthma are especially susceptible to its effects, they should take special precautions during periods of increased air pollution.

Allergenic Extracts Allergenic extracts contain allergenic materials that are used in the diagnosis and treatment of allergic people. These extracts are prepared by: (1) grinding and defatting the material; (2) extracting the allergenic component into an extraction fluid, usually buffered saline; (3) dialyzing the extract; and (4) sterilizing the end product. Two common methods of standardizing an allergenic extract are weight by volume and protein nitrogen unit. Neither of these methods may necessarily reflect the true allergenic potency of the extract.

Weight by volume (wt/v) is the amount of dry material in a given volume of extracting fluid; for example, a 1:10 dilution is prepared from 10 grams of material in 100 milliliters (ml) of extracting fluid. Protein nitrogen unit (PNU) is the nitrogen content of the protein in an extract. The extracts used for skin tests by the prick or the scratch method are usually prepared 1:10 to 1:20 weight by volume in 50 percent glycerin, and for intradermal testing, 1:1,000 weight by volume or 400 to 1,000 PNU/ml. Allergenic extracts lose their potency over time or, especially, at higher temperatures. For this reason, they should always be refrigerated. The extracts used in immunotherapy are prepared at several levels of increasing dilution; treatment begins with a dilute solution, and gradually the quantity and concentration are increased.

Allpyral is another type of allergenic extract used in immunotherapy. This extract is prepared by a different method, one designed to slow the rate of allergenic absorption following injection of the extract into a patient. The allergenic materials are extracted along with the organic solvent pyridine; then the solution is precipitated by alum. After removal of the excess pyridine and alum, the allergenic precipitate is again suspended in saline. The advantages of using allpyral extracts are, first, that fewer injections are needed and, second, that larger amounts of allergenic materials can be administered, with the lesser risk of allergic reaction. The main drawback is the uncertainty about the efficacy of the extract; it has not been clearly established that allpyral extracts are as effective as conventional allergenic ones. Several newer allergenic extracts may be marketed in the near future. Among these are the so-called gluteraldahyde-linked polymerized type, which induce a good protective immune response with less allergic side effects. They also require considerably fewer injections.

Allergens   Allergens are a special type of antigen that are responsible for clinical symptoms in allergic people. Antigens are foreign substances that induce an immune response in normal individuals. A person may be exposed to an allergen by inhalation, ingestion, or penetration of the skin. Allergens that are inhaled can be of either indoor or outdoor varieties, although the two environments appear to be intimately related.

The allergenic particles in *outdoor* allergens are derived mainly from components of plants that are widely dispersed by wind. Examples of these particles are plant pollen, spores from fungi, actinomycetes, bacteria, mosses, and ferns. Their composition varies by region, which, in turn, is influenced by, among other things, climate, cycles of plant growth, wind, temperature variations, rain, and agricultural activities. The major outdoor allergens consist of plant pollen and fungal spores. Descriptions of these allergens may be found under separate headings.

Indoor allergens occur primarily in the home and the workplace. The most important allergens in this category are house dust, mites, animal danders, feathers, mold spores, and pollen. The indoor environment is affected by air-conditioning and heating systems, by humidifiers, people's personal habits, and their hobbies. The work environment is affected by such factors as smoking, the type of job or industry, degree of ventilation and humidification. A person's occupation may be the only source of exposure to the allergens responsible for his or her symptoms. It is becoming increasingly important to study occupations as a potential source of allergens. Respiratory symptoms associated with an occupation may be caused by an allergy or by an irritant effect on the respiratory tract.

Some industrial materials are also known to cause asthma on an allergic basis. Among these are:

MATERIAL	INDUSTRY
Serum from animals, birds, fish, or insects; danders; animal secretions; animal excreta; contaminated water	Veterinary medicine; animal husbandry; poultry breeding; laboratory work; fishing; sericulture
Castor beans; green coffee beans; papain; pancreatic extracts; organic dusts; molds	Vegetable oil and food

MATERIAL	INDUSTRY
Flour	Baking; farming; grain handling
Bacillus subtilis enzymes; hog trypsin	Detergents; certain medications and food additives
Ethylenediamine; phthalic anhydride; trimellitic anhydride; certain isocyanates	Plastics; rubber; resins
Phenylglycine acid chloride; sulphone chloramides; antibiotics	Pharmaceutical manufacturing
Complex salts of platinum	Metal refining
Plicatic acid	Wood processing (western red cedar)

Allergic (IgE) Antibodies   Allergic (IgE) antibodies are the antibodies responsible for atopic allergic reactions. Minute quantities of IgE antibodies can be detected in almost everyone, but high concentrations are usually found in atopic patients with allergic asthma or hay fever. The tendency to produce allergic antibodies in response to common environmental substances, or allergens, is characteristic of atopic patients. Such responses are currently believed to be under genetic control. *See also* Antibodies.

Allergic Bronchopulmonary Aspergillosis   Abbreviated ABPA, this is an unusual lung disease found in allergic asthmatics and caused by an allergic reaction to a fungus growing in the bronchial tubes. Patients with this form of asthma characteristically have episodes of patchy pneumonia in their lungs and high levels of IgE and eosinophils. *See also* Aspergillus.

Allergic Conjunctivitis   Allergic conjunctivitis is a common allergic reaction of the eyes. The most prominent symptom is itchy, watery eyes and a red lining on the whites of the eyes. Allergic conjunctivitis is often associated with other allergic symptoms such as hay fever, but sometimes it is the only complaint. Symptomatic treatment with antihistaminics produces significant improvement in most cases. In severe cases, allergic evaluation and treatment is carried out in the usual manner, that is, by skin testing and eosinophil and IgE quantification.

Allergic Rhinitis   Commonly known as hay fever, allergic rhinitis is a complex of symptoms characterized by attacks of sneezing, a runny stuffy nose and postnasal drip, frequent eye irritation, and ear congestion resulting from specific allergic reactions. These symptoms may be limited to one season of the year or they may be perennial, depending on the presence of a specific allergen in the local environment. Severe nasal obstruction may occur, which can interfere with normal sinus drainage and with the openings of the Eustachian tubes, producing headaches, impaired hearing, and secondary sinus and ear infections. During the allergy season, it is not unusual for a person to complain of fatigue, irritability, and a loss of well-being. Not everyone who has nasal symptoms, however, is suffering from allergic rhinitis.

Allergist An allergist is a medical doctor certified by the American Board of Allergy and Immunology who specializes in the diagnosis and treatment of allergies.

Allergoids Allergoids are allergenic materials that have been modified in such a way that the allergenic activity ceases but the ability to induce antibody formation is retained. In theory, an allergic patient can receive a much higher dose of an allergenic extract without risking an allergic reaction. This type of allergenic extract may be the material used for immunotherapy in the future.

Allergy The word *allergy,* from the Greek *allos* ("other") and *ergeon* ("action"), was coined in 1906 by Baron Clemens von Pirquet, who recognized that the introduction of a foreign substance into a tissue can alter the tissue's capacity to react to a subsequent encounter with the same substance. Von Pirquet discovered that this altered response is both protective (that is, it is an immune response) and potentially harmful (that is, it can cause a person to become hypersensitive). Since von Pirquet's time, physicians and researchers have redefined the term, and it is today synonymous with *hypersensitivity.* Many allergists prefer the restricted meaning: "hypersensitivity reactions caused by allergic antibodies."

Alveoli Alveoli are the tiny air sacs in the lungs.

Anaphylaxis The word *anaphylaxis* was coined to describe a condition opposite to that of protection, or *prophylaxis.* Clinically, it is characterized by symptoms that occur within a few minutes to a few hours after exposure to a substance, or allergen, against which a patient produces specific allergic antibodies. Symptoms are attributed to the release of various pharmacological substances such as histamine from target cells after an allergen-antibody reaction. Systemic manifestations are: generalized urticaria (hives); angioedema (swelling); bronchospasm (wheezing); hypotension (low blood pressure); and diarrhea. Symptoms vary in intensity from person to person, and extremely severe attacks can be fatal if they are not treated promptly.

In the past, horse antiserum was the most frequent cause of ana-phylaxis. At one time or another, however, almost every substance has been implicated as a cause of an anaphylactic reaction—including antibiotics, hormones, diagnostic agents, animal serum, insect venom, enzymes, local anesthetics, and foods. During the 1970s, penicillin was identified as probably the most common cause, followed by reactions to venom from insect stings of the order Hymenoptera, for example, bees, wasps, and yellow jackets. Some common foods that can cause anaphylaxis are nuts, especially peanuts; shellfish; eggs; and berries.

A common method of administering antigen that induces anaphylactic reactions is parenterally (the introduction of a substance into the body by means other than oral), whether intravenously, intramuscularly, subcutaneously, or intradermally. Treating an anaphylactic reaction clinically requires prompt parenteral administration of adrenalin and antihistaminics. It is more effective in the long run, however, to identify the offending substance and prevent future exposure to it.

Angioedema　Angioedema is a localized swelling of the deeper layers of the skin. In contrast, an urticarial reaction occurs in the superficial areas of the skin. In angioedema, the swelling often involves the eyelids, lips, hands, or feet. Swelling usually lasts a few hours and seldom more than twenty-four. Because they appear to have similar mechanisms, angioedema and urticaria are ordinarily studied together.

Angioedema, Hereditary　Hereditary angiodema is a rare, inherited disorder due to a deficiency of a normally occurring blood protein that inhibits the complement system. The disease produces recurrent abdominal pain and episodes of swelling, mostly in the face and extremities or in the air passages. It can be fatal if swelling, which occurs in the tongue, throat, or larynx, shuts off air to the lungs.

Antibiotic　An antibiotic is a substance produced by certain bacteria or by chemical synthesis that, even in small amounts, can kill other bacteria.

Antibodies　Antibodies are substances produced in response to a foreign substance (antigen) that are capable of reacting with that particular antigen. Antibodies are contained in a special type of protein called an immunoglobulin, which is produced by specialized "plasma" cells. Antibody activity in the serum is confined to a hetero- geneous group of gamma globulin molecules. Antibodies belong to one of five immunoglobulin classes: (1) immunoglobulin G (IgG); (2) immunoglobulin A (IgA); (3) immunoglobulin M (IgM); (4) immunoglobulin D (IgD); or (5) immunoglobulin E (IgE). They are an important part of the defense, or immune, mechanism, which, in turn, is essential to survival. Under certain conditions, antibodies may cause allergic tissue damage, called hypersensitivity reaction (*see also* hypersensitivity). The antibodies responsible for hypersensitivity re- actions of the allergic type, such as hay fever and asthma, belong to the IgE class. *See also* Immunoglobulins.

Antibodies, Blocking   A blocking antibody is an antibody of one class that combines with an antigen, thus preventing the antigen from re- acting with an antibody of another class.

Anticholinergic   *See* Bronchodilator.

Antigens   Antigens are foreign substances that are capable of induc- ing an immune response in normal individuals. Most of the naturally occurring antigens are large molecules and, more frequently, pro- teins, although high-molecular-weight polysaccharides (sugars) are also potent antigens. An immune response consists of a humoral re- sponse mediated by antibodies and a cellular immune response medi- ated by mononuclear cells. *See also* Allergens.

Table 2.1.   **Frequency of Aspirin Intolerance under Various Conditions**

TYPE OF POPULATION	PERCENTAGE
Chronic urticaria	23.2
Asthma	3.8
Rhinitis	1.4
Normal	0.9

Antihistamine   An antihistamine is a drug used to neutralize or in- hibit the action of histamine; antihistamines are divided into six classes in the treatment of allergic disorders: ethanolamines, ethylene- diamines, alkylamines, piperazines, and phenothiazines; the sixth class is a group of miscellaneous compounds.

Antiserum   Antiserum is serum that contains antibodies. It may be prepared in animals by immunization with a specific antigen, or it may be isolated from humans previously exposed to the antigen. Animal antiserums were often used in the past for treating infections; today, their use is limited to antisera against snake venom and other potent toxins and antilymphocyte serum, which is used in organ transplants.

Human antiserum is frequently used for the prevention of certain infections such as infectious hepatitis. Antiserums prepared for use against toxins are called antitoxins.

Arachidonic Acid   Arachidonic acid is a fatty acid that may be broken down in the body to produce substances that are very important in the production of asthma. Among these are the cyclooxygenase products (certain prostaglandins and thromboxane), some of which can induce important bronchial spasms or asthma in several species, including man and others, such as PGE2, which can actually open the breathing tubes and may help in the future treatment of asthma.

Other arachidonic acid products—called SRS-A leukotrienes and referred to as LTC4, LTD4, and LTE4—induce powerful bronchial spasms or asthmatic responses, particularly in the very small breathing tubes. Overall, it is thought that leukotriene components of SRS-A play a very important role in atopic asthma. Still other lipooxygenase products of arachidonic acid are important, in that they act as powerful attractants for certain white blood cells in the skin and other tissues.

Asbestosis   Asbestosis is a chronic inflammation of the lungs caused by inhaled asbestos fibers.

Aspergillus   Aspergillus is a genus of fungi that belongs to the class Fungi Imperfecti. Several species are saprophytic; that is, they obtain food by absorbing dissolved organic material. They may cause allergic reactions, however, such as asthma and hay fever in sensitized persons. Aspergillus can also grow in the lungs, producing a tumorlike mass called an aspergilloma. Still another condition associated with this fungus is a disease called pulmonary allergic aspergillosis. Patients with this condition have symptoms of asthma, highly elevated levels of allergic (IgE) antibodies, and specific IgE and IgG antibodies against the aspergillus, plus eosinophilea. *See also* Allergic bronchopulmonary aspergillus; Fungi.

Aspirin-Induced Asthma   This is a special category of intrinsic asthma induced by the ingestion of aspirin. It may occur as a triad of asthma, nasal polyps, and increased eosinophils, associated with severe potentially fatal reactions to aspirin. Aspirin intolerance can also be associated with chronic urticaria (see Table 2.1). The cause of aspirin-induced asthma may involve arachidonic acid, since aspirin may inhibit its cyclooxygenase products (*see* Arachidonic Acid) and allow selective breaking down of arachidonic acid via the lipooxygenase pathway.

Asthma   Asthma is a disease that is characterized by recurrent episodes of difficult breathing and by wheezing, with periods of nearly complete freedom from symptoms. The episodes of difficulty are due to a narrowing of the bronchial tubes, swelling of the bronchial walls, and increased mucus production. Asthma symptoms may be sporadic and mild, they may occur frequently in spells of fluctuating severity, or they may become continuous and incapacitating. A variety of factors may induce an asthmatic attack in a susceptible person:

Immunological   These factors are allergens that can induce asthma attacks in allergic patients (*see also* Allergens).

Nonimmunological   Viral respiratory infections, aspirin and related drugs, weather, air pollution, inhaled irritants, emotional responses, and exercise, among other factors, can influence or precipitate asthma attacks.

Respiratory infections are among the most common causes of asthma attacks. Recent studies have shown that respiratory viruses are capable of causing asthma, but there is considerable doubt that bacterial infections play a significant role in the production of asthma. In the past, it was suggested that asthma symptoms are related to bacterial allergy, and patients were frequently treated with bacterial vaccines. Today, most authorities are of the opinion that bacterial allergy is not a frequent cause of asthma; therefore, immunotherapy using bacterial vaccines has, for the most part, been abandoned.

Concerning the psychological factors involved, much has been written about the role of emotion in asthma and other allergies, but no convincing evidence exists that psychogenic factors actually cause allergies as such. On the other hand, there is little doubt that emotional factors can precipitate asthma attacks or aggravate allergies. Conversely, psychiatric disturbances may result from a chronic incapacitating condition such as asthma that is not treated properly. For these reasons, patients with severe allergies, like many patients with other chronic, incapacitating diseases, may require psychiatric counseling.

See also Bacterial Allergy.

Asthma, Extrinsic   Extrinsic asthma is a seasonal form of asthma caused by allergens found in the environment.

Asthma, Intrinsic   Intrinsic asthma is a nonseasonal form of asthma caused by respiratory infection or by other precipitating factors, not by allergies.

Asthma, Mixed   Mixed asthma is a form of asthma caused by both extrinsic-allergy and intrinsic-nonallergic factors.

Atopic   *Atopic* means having an inherited tendency to suffer from allergic diseases.

Atopic Dermatitis   Atopic dermatitis is characterized by chronically itchy, superficially inflamed skin, often accompanied by allergic symptoms such as hay fever and asthma. It also occurs in patients whose families have histories of allergies. The disease frequently occurs on the face and at or near the elbows and knees. Although atopic dermatitis is associated with allergies, the skin lesions do not have an allergic mechanism in most patients. Symptoms are commonly worse during the cold part of the year and are aggravated by contact irritants. In some people, skin symptoms appear to be aggravated in part by certain foods or by exposure to inhaled allergens such as pollen.

Atopy   Over the years, *atopy* (from the Greek *atopia,* for "uncommonness") has been given various meanings. Broadly, it is a group of allergic diseases—mainly allergic rhinitis, allergic asthma, and some forms of eczema—that have some characteristics in common. Among these characteristics are a frequent, positive family history of similar allergic illnesses and the presence of increased serum levels of allergic antibodies to such common environmental allergens as pollen, molds, house dust, and animal danders. The most common feature of atopy in atopic patients is the tendency to develop allergic antibodies to common inhalant substances as a result of natural exposure. This tendency is now believed to be genetically determined.

Autoimmune Diseases   Also called autoallergic diseases, autoimmune diseases result when a person's immune system reacts against its own tissues and organs.

B Cells   B cells, or B lymphocytes, are lymphocytes derived from the bone marrow. They are involved in the production of antibodies.

Bacterial Allergy   Infections can play an important role in allergic disorders. People with asthma often have increased symptoms following infections of the respiratory tract, whereas people with allergic rhinitis and asthma appear to have an increased incidence of respiratory infections. In the past, many allergists felt that the increased symptoms associated with infections were caused by allergy to bacterial products, so patients were treated with bacterial vaccines. The effectiveness of this type of treatment remains controversial. Most of the studies showing the beneficial effects of bacterial extracts have been based on clinical observations rather than sound experimental data. Recent studies clearly show that viral, rather than bacterial, agents are the microorganisms responsible for respiratory infections that precipitate asthma symptoms.

There is no evidence that bacterial allergy causes asthma symptoms, nor that bacterial vaccines are effective in treating the disease. Viral infections, however, can precipitate asthma symptoms, though probably not by an allergic mechanism.

Bagassosis   Bagassosis is a form of allergic lung disorder caused by exposure to moldy sugar cane fiber. *See also* Hypersensitivity Pneumonitis.

Basophil   A basophil is a type of white cell that circulates in the blood. Cells of this type have surface receptors for the allergic (IgE) antibodies and participate actively in an allergic reaction. Upon exposure to an allergen, the reaction between the allergen and the antibodies on the surface of the cell initiates a series of intracellular events that culminate in the release of histamine and other chemicals responsible for allergic symptoms.

Blood Groups   Blood groups are categories of blood determined by inherited antigens present on red blood cell surfaces. The most important blood groups are A, B, AB, and O; it is these groups that are referred to in speaking of "incompatible" blood.

Bronchiectasis   Bronchiectasis is a disease in which dilations occur in the air passages of the lungs, often as a result of a long-standing infection.

Bronchodilator   A bronchodilator is medication that causes bronchodilation (relaxation of the bronchial muscles). It is administered orally, intravenously, by inhalation, or by injection.

Bronchospasm Bronchospasm is spasmodic tightening of the muscles surrounding the bronchial tubes.

Carotid Body Carotid bodies are small organs present in the neck. They have a protective function, which is to respond to rapid drops in the oxygen level and to increases in the carbon dioxide level. Resection of the carotid bodies, called glomectomy, was once promoted as treatment for asthma; controlled studies, however, did not show significant improvement after surgery, and the treatment has been abandoned.

Cascade Reaction A cascade reaction is a series of reactions, such as that of the serum complement system, in which the reaction of the first component triggers the reaction of the next component, and so on, until all components of the system have reacted.

Challenge Test A challenge test is a medical procedure, also known as provocative testing, used to identify substances to which a person is sensitive by deliberately exposing the person to diluted amounts of the substance; a positive bronchial challenge is one in which pulmonary function decreases. *See* Inhalation Challenge.

Cholinergic Urticaria Cholinergic urticaria is a special type of urticaria, or hives, characterized by small, short-term wheals (welts that form suddenly) that develop in response to a combination of factors, including exercise, heat, and emotional stress. Exercise is the most frequent precipitating factor. Cholinergic hives occur most often in the upper limbs and do not have an immunological mechanism.

Climate and Allergies Climate is a combination of many meteorological forces, including temperature, wind velocity, barometric pressure, and humidity. It strongly affects allergens in the environment, such as pollen, mold, and air pollutants—particularly their concentration and dispersal. For this reason, climate may have a marked effect on people with respiratory allergies. Pollen-producing plants that grow in a given region do so because of the region's climate. Ragweed, for example, is the most prominent hay-fever-producing plant in many parts of the United States, but it is not found in the Pacific west or in southern Florida. Warm, humid climates favor the growth of molds. It has long been established that climate affects the concentration of particles in the air, including allergens. For instance, during periods of thermal inversion, there is a marked increase in the amount of pol-

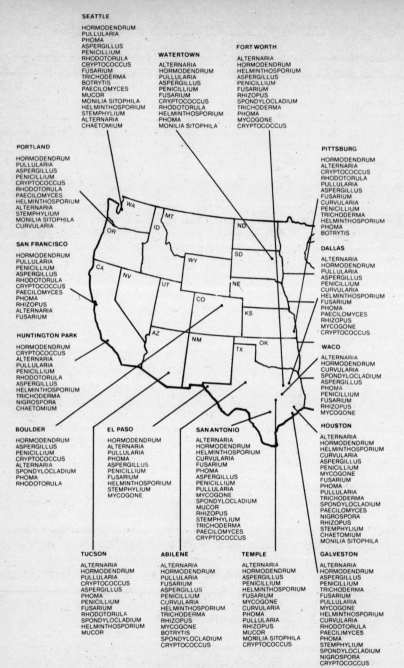

SEATTLE
HORMODENDRUM
PULLULARIA
PHOMA
ASPERGILLUS
PENICILLIUM
RHODOTORULA
CRYPTOCOCCUS
FUSARIUM
TRICHODERMA
BOTRYTIS
PAECILOMYCES
MUCOR
MONILIA SITOPHILA
HELMINTHOSPORIUM
STEMPHYLIUM
ALTERNARIA
CHAETOMIUM

WATERTOWN
ALTERNARIA
HORMODENDRUM
PULLULARIA
ASPERGILLUS
PENICILLIUM
FUSARIUM
CRYPTOCOCCUS
RHODOTORULA
HELMINTHOSPORIUM
PHOMA
MONILIA SITOPHILA

FORT WORTH
ALTERNARIA
HORMODENDRUM
HELMINTHOSPORIUM
ASPERGILLUS
PENICILLIUM
FUSARIUM
RHIZOPUS
SPONDYLOCLADIUM
TRICHODERMA
PHOMA
MYCOGONE
CRYPTOCOCCUS

PORTLAND
HORMODENDRUM
PULLULARIA
ASPERGILLUS
PENICILLIUM
CRYPTOCOCCUS
RHODOTORULA
PAECILOMYCES
HELMINTHOSPORIUM
ALTERNARIA
STEMPHYLIUM
MONILIA SITOPHILA
CURVULARIA

PITTSBURG
HORMODENDRUM
ALTERNARIA
CRYPTOCOCCUS
RHODOTORULA
PULLULARIA
ASPERGILLUS
FUSARIUM
CURVULARIA
PENICILLIUM
TRICHODERMA
HELMINTHOSPORIUM
PHOMA
BOTRYTIS

SAN FRANCISCO
HORMODENDRUM
PULLULARIA
PENICILLIUM
ASPERGILLUS
RHODOTORULA
CRYPTOCOCCUS
PAECILOMYCES
PHOMA
RHIZOPUS
ALTERNARIA
FUSARIUM

DALLAS
ALTERNARIA
HORMODENDRUM
PULLULARIA
ASPERGILLUS
PENICILLIUM
CURVULARIA
HELMINTHOSPORIUM
FUSARIUM
PHOMA
PAECILOMYCES
RHIZOPUS
MYCOGONE
CRYPTOCOCCUS

HUNTINGTON PARK
HORMODENDRUM
CRYPTOCOCCUS
ALTERNARIA
PULLULARIA
PENICILLIUM
RHODOTORULA
ASPERGILLUS
HELMINTHOSPORIUM
TRICHODERMA
NIGROSPORA
CHAETOMIUM

WACO
ALTERNARIA
HORMODENDRUM
CURVULARIA
SPONDYLOCLADIUM
ASPERGILLUS
PHOMA
PENICILLIUM
FUSARIUM
RHIZOPUS
MYCOGONE

BOULDER
HORMODENDRUM
ASPERGILLUS
PENICILLIUM
CRYPTOCOCCUS
ALTERNARIA
SPONDYLOCLADIUM
PHOMA
RHODOTORULA

EL PASO
HORMODENDRUM
ALTERNARIA
PULLULARIA
PHOMA
ASPERGILLUS
PENICILLIUM
FUSARIUM
HELMINTHOSPORIUM
STEMPHYLIUM
MYCOGONE

SAN ANTONIO
ALTERNARIA
HORMODENDRUM
HELMINTHOSPORIUM
CURVULARIA
FUSARIUM
PHOMA
ASPERGILLUS
PENICILLIUM
PULLULARIA
MYCOGONE
SPONDYLOCLADIUM
MUCOR
RHIZOPUS
STEMPHYLIUM
TRICHODERMA
PAECILOMYCES
CRYPTOCOCCUS

HOUSTON
ALTERNARIA
HORMODENDRUM
HELMINTHOSPORIUM
CURVULARIA
ASPERGILLUS
PENICILLIUM
MYCOGONE
FUSARIUM
PHOMA
PULLULARIA
TRICHODERMA
SPONDYLOCLADIUM
PAECILOMYCES
NIGROSPORA
RHIZOPUS
STEMPHYLIUM
CHAETOMIUM
MONILIA SITOPHILA

TUCSON
ALTERNARIA
HORMODENDRUM
PULLULARIA
CRYPTOCOCCUS
ASPERGILLUS
PHOMA
PENICILLIUM
FUSARIUM
RHODOTORULA
SPONDYLOCLADIUM
HELMINTHOSPORIUM
MUCOR

ABILENE
ALTERNARIA
HORMODENDRUM
PULLULARIA
FUSARIUM
ASPERGILLUS
PENICILLIUM
CURVULARIA
HELMINTHOSPORIUM
TRICHODERMA
RHIZOPUS
MYCOGONE
BOTRYTIS
SPONDYLOCLADIUM
CRYPTOCOCCUS

TEMPLE
ALTERNARIA
HORMODENDRUM
ASPERGILLUS
PENICILLIUM
HELMINTHOSPORIUM
FUSARIUM
MYCOGONE
CURVULARIA
PHOMA
PULLULARIA
RHIZOPUS
MUCOR
MONILIA SITOPHILA
CRYPTOCOCCUS

GALVESTON
ALTERNARIA
HORMODENDRUM
ASPERGILLUS
PENICILLIUM
TRICHODERMA
FUSARIUM
PULLULARIA
MYCOGONE
HELMINTHOSPORIUM
CURVULARIA
RHODOTORULA
PAECILIMYCES
PHOMA
STEMPHYLIUM
SPONDYLOCLADIUM
NIGROSPORA
CRYPTOCOCCUS

Maps showing the dominant aerobiological populations in the order of their frequency of occurrence at different monitoring stations.

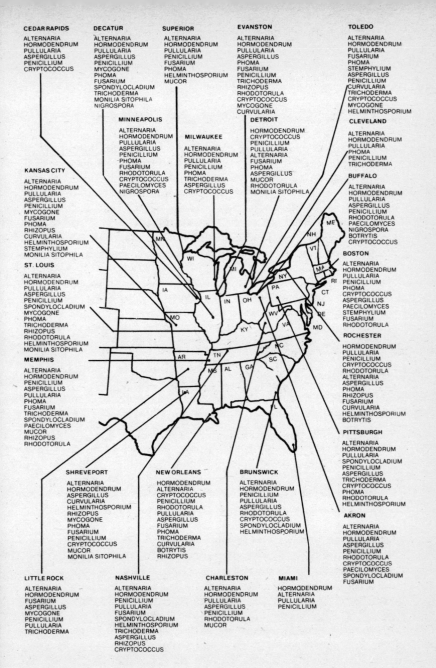

Adapted from material originally appearing in *Annals of Allergy*, vol. 22, pp. 578–79, November 1964; copyright © 1964.

lutants in the air. These pollutants are associated with deleterious health effects, especially among people with respiratory problems.

Climate Therapy A change of climate is one of the oldest treatments known, having been a recommended treatment since ancient times. In theory, a dry climate with low air pollution and vegetation that produces a small amount of pollen should benefit someone with allergic symptoms who is sensitive to pollen and molds. Some medical evidence suggests that some patients who change climate will show improvement; but changing climate is not necessarily followed by beneficial results. In fact, such a change occasionally induces the development of new allergies. The multiplicity of meteorological and environmental factors in climates, and the marked variability of patients' responses to these factors, make it virtually impossible to prescribe a favorable climate for a particular patient. When a change of climate is prescribed (as it sometimes is in severe cases), a trial period of several months in the new climate is usually recommended before the transfer becomes permanent. That way, more can be learned about the effect of the new climate on a person, enabling a physician to suggest another climate if the original one is not suitable.

Cold Urticaria Cold urticaria is the occurrence of hives precipitated by exposure to cold; often this condition is associated with an underlying disease.

Complement Complement is a group of proteins, many of which are enzymes that interact sequentially after activation by an antigen-antibody reaction. Complement plays an important mediatory role in immune reactions by helping attract cells to the area, by increasing the permeability of the blood vessels, and by causing lysis (destruction) of the attacking microorganisms. Under certain conditions, however, the complement system may also play a part in hypersensitivity reactions such as serum sickness.

Contact Dermatitis Contact dermatitis is a type of reaction in which local areas of the skin become inflamed upon contact with certain substances. The area of skin itches, turns red, and may break out in papules, or blisters. In time, the lesions thicken and crack, and the skin changes color. Usually, a well-defined border develops between the affected area and the normal skin. The causative agent may act as an irritant or as a sensitizer, inducing delayed allergic reactions. Delayed contact allergy is not mediated by allergic antibodies, as it is in hay fever; instead, the allergy is produced by certain sensitized cells (lymphocytes) in response to an antigen, the substance that causes the irritation. The antigens responsible for contact allergy are usually small (in terms of molecular weight) chemicals that must first combine with local proteins before becoming antigens.

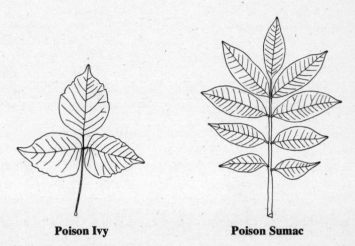

Poison Ivy   **Poison Sumac**

Poison ivy, metals, cosmetics, and drugs are common causative agents. Poison ivy belongs to the plant family Anacardiaseae and is the most common cause of contact allergy. The material that causes the reaction is an oil resin called urushiol, found in the sap of the plant. Skin reactions vary in severity from mild lesions to severe lesions that require treatment using steroids (cortisone). In highly sensitive persons who have come in contact with poison ivy, immunotherapy has been tried; but the treatment has not yet been demonstrated as effective. Other members of the poison ivy family are eastern poison oak, western poison oak, and poison sumac.

Among metals, nickel, mercury, and chromates are common sensitizers. Most commercial metals are contaminated by other metals, particularly nickel. For example, it is common for someone sensitive to nickel who comes in contact with a chrome-plated object to have a skin reaction.

The incidence of contact allergy to cosmetics is low. Probably the most common allergic reaction to cosmetics is to the chemical paraphenylenediamine, a basic ingredient in oxidation-type permanent hair dyes. Sun-screening lotions, perfumes, and lipsticks are among the cosmetics frequently associated with contact allergy.

Among drugs, by far the most common skin sensitizer is the antibiotic neomycin, which is used as an antibiotic cream. Penicillin and antihistaminic creams are also frequent causes of contact allergy. Ethylenediamine, a chemical often used as a stabilizer in many topical drugs, is a potent sensitizer and is the cause of numerous reactions to topically administered medications.

Contrast Media Reactions   Contrast media reactions are adverse reactions to iodinated dyes injected during certain x-ray studies. Adverse reactions to contrast media occur frequently, with the incidence estimated at 1 in 1,000. Reactions may take the form of hives, laryngeal obstruction, bronchospasm, or, in severe cases, shock and death. The symptoms are similar to those of anaphylaxis, although current evidence suggests that this reaction is not immunologically mediated.

Cortisone   Also called corticosteroid, cortisone is a hormone produced by the adrenal gland or made synthetically. Sometimes it is used in treating allergic diseases. Although effective, cortisone has side effects, such as weight gain. Topical corticosteroids are applied to the skin to reduce the inflammation of eczema.

Cromolyn Sodium   Cromolyn sodium is the generic name for a medication used to treat asthma; it is marketed under the brand name Intal and is given in the form of an inhaled powder.

Cross-Reactivity   Cross-reactivity is a condition in which the body mistakes one compound for another of similar or identical chemical composition. Thus antigens or allergens that cross-react with one another always share some common chemical structure or group.

Cyclooxygenase products   *See* Arachidonic Acid.

Cytotoxic Food Tests   Cytotoxic food tests are tests in which a person's white cells are used to diagnose an allergy. In the test, the white cells are incubated for a given period with an extract of the suspect food or inhalant. After incubation, the white cells are examined to determine whether any changes have occurred. Numerous technical difficulties are involved in administering this test. In addition, reports in which the test has been subjected to rigid experimental study have failed to demonstrate the validity of this type of test.

Danders   Next to house dust, animal danders are the most common nonseasonal, inhaled allergen. Animal danders may induce hay fever and asthma symptoms, or they may produce skin reactions such as urticaria. The allergy usually becomes obvious to the patient or the patient's family, but in some cases the relationship between allergic symptoms and exposure to animals is not readily apparent. It is also important to realize that the animal need not be present at the time the symptoms occur, since animal danders and hair may contaminate the house environment over a considerable period of time. Of the animal danders, cat dander is the most common cause of dander allergy. Variations in allergens among different breeds of cat has been suggested, although this is only a theory at present. Dog dander is also a common cause of allergies, and allergic responses to various dog breeds have been demonstrated experimentally.

Because the major allergens are present in the epidermal scales and not in the hair, both long-haired and short-haired dogs cause allergic symptoms. In assessing sensitivity to a house pet, a trial period of removing the animal and extensive cleaning may be necessary before clinical sensitivity can be established. Allergic reactions to horsehair are less of a problem today, with the decreased use of horses and horsehair products such as mattress and furniture padding. Besides cats, dogs, and horses, a number of other pets and farm animals—for example, hamsters, rabbits, guinea pigs, and birds—can cause allergic problems. Guinea pigs are known to possess powerful allergens, which can cause allergies in individuals who are exposed to guinea pig dander over long periods of time.

Avoidance of animal dander or danders is, at the moment, the best treatment available. In general, people who are allergic to animal danders should avoid keeping pets at home and should not acquire new pets, since there is a good chance of their becoming sensitized to the new animals. A recent well-controlled study has demonstrated a good response to immunotherapy, using a cat pelt extract for treating asthma in a group of cat-sensitive patients.

Decongestant   A decongestant is any of a group of drugs used primarily in the treatment of hay fever, vasomotor rhinitis, and intrinsic rhinitis.

Dermatitis Herpetiformis   Dermatitis herpetiformis is a chronic, debilitating, immunologically mediated skin disorder characterized by firm blisters with reddened bases.

Dermographism   Dermographism is increased sensitivity of the skin to stroking, characterized by the appearance of a wheal and by redness of the skin. It is the mechanism for urticarial lesions that develop on the parts of the body where clothing is tight, for example, body areas underneath brassieres or belts. Dermographism, which appears a few minutes after the skin is scraped by a sharp object, is common, occurring in 5 to 10 percent of the population. It does not, however, appear to be associated with allergies, although it sometimes appears in patients suffering from hives.

Desensitization   *See* Hyposensitization.

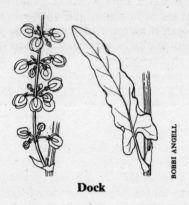

BOBBI ANGELL

Dock

Dock and Knotweed Family   Dock and knotweed plants are common in acid soil throughout North America. They are mainly of local importance as causes of hay fever.

Drug Allergy   A drug allergy is an adverse reaction to a drug or medication that occurs as a consequence of interaction between that drug and the patient's immune system. The term *drug allergy* is frequently used to indicate the undesirable effect of a drug. Most adverse reactions, however, are not allergic reactions. Other mechanisms are:

> *toxic effect*—drugs which, when given to patients in sufficient dosage, can have an adverse effect
> *side effect*—effects related to the biologic properties of a drug, for example, drowsiness from antihistamines
> *idiosyncrasy*—a mysterious, unusual susceptibility to a drug.

Drug allergies are less common in children than in adults. At the same time, there is no convincing evidence that drug allergy is more common in allergic (atopic) patients who are sensitive to common inhaled pollens and molds. A drug allergy can be caused by such immunological mechanisms as anaphylaxis; serum, or drug, sickness; and contact allergy.

Anaphylaxis is a severe allergic reaction that produces symptoms which may include generalized hives; bronchospasm (difficulty in breathing); decreased blood pressure; and, in severe cases, shock and death. The reaction occurs most often after an injection of a medication. Penicillin is the drug that most frequently causes an anaphylactic reaction; others are hormones, other antibiotics, and analgesics (painkillers).

In the type of reaction known as serum sickness, such symptoms as fever, hives, and painful joints occur six to eight days after the administration of large amounts of a serum or a drug. A few of the drugs that cause this type of allergic reaction are: penicillin; sulfas; phenytoin (a drug used for epilepsy); and propyl thiouracil (used to treat an overactive thyroid condition). Serum sickness is so named because this reaction was originally described in patients receiving foreign serum such as horse serum. Today, drugs are more common causes of the reaction.

Drug fever occurs several days after a drug is administered, and disappears rapidly when the medication is discontinued. Penicillin and other antibiotics, as well as barbiturates, are a common cause of this type of reaction.

Anaphylaxis and several types of inflammatory reaction may involve the lungs, producing an adverse reaction. Patients who inhale pituitary powder, for example, may exhibit symptoms of hypersensitivity pneumonitis similar to farmer's lung. A type of eosinophilic pneumonia has been linked to penicillin, sulfas, and some other drugs. Allergic reactions that produce inflammation and fibrosis of the lungs have been observed in patients who were given nitrofurantoin or certain sulfas.

Skin reactions are common and may take the form of hives, angioedema (generalized swelling), eczema, or blisters. Antibiotic creams, particularly those containing neomycin, are known to produce contact allergies. An extremely severe type of skin reaction, called exfoliative dermatitis or Stevens-Johnson syndrome, which can result from the use of any of a number of drugs, is characterized by generalized redness, itching, and peeling of the skin.

Other adverse reactions may involve the liver, kidneys, or blood. Many such reactions can be severe and are potentially life-threatening, especially when they affect the production of white blood cells, red blood cells, and platelets.

Diagnosis of drug allergy is usually made clinically, since no laboratory or skin tests are available for most drugs other than penicillin. Treatment is based on discontinuing use of drugs. In severe cases, the patient may be treated with corticosteroids (cortisone).

Drugs Used in Treating Allergies Following is a list of drugs commonly used to treat allergies:

Adrenalin (epinephrine) A hormone produced by the adrenal glands. As a drug, it is used in the treatment of severe acute allergic reactions such as anaphylaxis and asthma. It is usually injected, although it can be administered by inhalation (see chapter 3, "Allergy Emergencies and How to Cope with Them").

Aminophyllin See theophylline below in this listing.

Antihistaminics Drugs used in treating allergic symptoms. The chemical structure of antihistaminics is similar to that of histamine: they act by blocking the action of histamine, a substance liberated during allergic reactions, which is responsible for many allergic symptoms. Antihistaminics are especially useful in treating nasal allergies, particularly sneezing and runny noses. Several chemical groups of antihistaminics are available, to which patients may have varying responses. Drowsiness is a common side effect of antihistaminics. Although the side effects are not serious, a change of medication in some patients may be necessary.

Beclomethasone An inhaled steroid (cortisone) used in the treatment of severe and chronic asthma. The main use of beclomethasone is in treating patients with chronic severe asthma who would otherwise have to be treated using oral cortisone. Its advantages are that it causes fewer steroid-induced side effects and can be given in relatively small doses.

Bronchodilators Drugs that relax the smooth muscle of constricted bronchi. The main use of bronchodilators is in treating asthma.

Cromolyn A drug used in the treatment of asthma. The effect of cromolyn is unique; it is not a bronchodilator, nor does it block any of the chemicals released during an allergic reaction. Instead, it appears to prevent the release of these chemicals following the antibody reaction on the surface of the sensitized basophils and mast cells.

Corticosteroids (cortisone) Hormones produced by the cortex, or outer part, of the adrenal glands. Corticosteroids are extremely useful in treating severe allergic reactions and can be given orally, topically, or by injection. The onset of their action, however, is delayed, which reduces their effectiveness in such acute life-threatening reactions as anaphylaxis.

Decadron A type of corticosteroid drug used in the treatment of severe allergies. It can be given intravenously, orally, or intramuscularly. A special preparation called decadron turbinaire, given by nasal inhalation, is often highly effective in treating nasal allergies that do not respond to conventional antihistaminic decongestive treatment.

Depo-Medrol A corticosteriod drug of sustained action that is administered intramuscularly. Depo-Medrol is occasionally used in treating patients with severe chronic allergies when tablets cannot be used.

Ephedrine A drug used in the treatment of asthma. Ephedrine is a component of numerous oral preparations in common use. With the recent appearance of more effective medications, the use of ephedrine has diminished.

Theophylline A group of xanthine derivatives used in the treatment of asthma. The most important effect of drugs in the theophylline group is their ability to relax smooth muscle, causing a dilation of the bronchial tubes, with an accompanying subsequent improvement of asthma symptoms. At one time, these drugs were commonly used in combination with other bronchodilators in single pills or were given intravenously in the case of severe asthma attacks. Recently, use of theophylline drugs has undergone a major revision as the preparation of these drugs has been improved and methods have been developed for measuring blood levels. Theophylline drugs are today recommended for the everyday treatment of asthma patients.

Ecology centers Ecology centers are controversial clinics or hospital units usually run by doctors who call themselves "clinical sociologists." According to their theories, many mysterious diseases involving a wide range of symptoms are attributable to allergic-type reactions to chemicals, pollutants, or to a long list of other substances found in minute quantities in the air, water, food, or general environment. Patients are often treated with exotic diets or in isolation rooms with specially filtered air and water and from which many synthetic materials have been removed.

There is no proof available from well-controlled double-blind studies to prove or disprove the benefit of treatment at these clinical ecology centers.

Eczema Eczema is an inflammation of the skin, marked by redness, itching, and scales.

Elimination (Provocative Challenge) Diets An elimination-challenge diet is a method of determining food allergens by temporarily and selectively eliminating common foods, especially those known to be allergenic, followed by ingestion of the suspected food allergens, one at a time, to see whether they will actually produce symptoms.

Emphysema Emphysema is a chronic disease of the lungs, in which the alveoli are permanently damaged or destroyed. It is typically characterized by difficult breathing and is associated with heavy, prolonged cigarette smoking.

Eosinophils Eosinophils are a type of white blood cell often found in greater numbers in the blood of patients with allergic diseases, as well as in the tissues of people who have had allergic reactions. Little is known about this type of cell, however. What *is* known about eosinophils is:\ they are attracted by a chemical released during an allergic reaction; they contain substances capable of neutralizing histamine and related chemical mediators, they probably play a role in regulating these reactions; because they contain a substance that is capable of damaging tissue.

Exercise Asthma Exercise can cause bronchospasm in asthmatic patients, particularly children. The changes that occur during an attack are the same as those in other types of asthma, but no immunological mechanism has yet been demonstrated. It is thought that inhalation of cold, dry air may contribute to the onset of the condition. Exercise-induced asthma can be prevented by pretreatment with one of the various medications used in treating asthma. Cromolyn and inhaled bronchodilators are especially useful for this purpose.

Exercise Urticaria Exercise urticaria is a newly described, potentially serious development of itchy hives, swelling, and, at times, collapse (anaphylactic shock) following such strenuous exercise as jogging. Such patients should carry Adrenalin kits and avoid overexertion, especially on hot days.

Extrinsic Asthma *See* Asthma, Extrinsic.

Farmer's Lung Farmer's lung is a form of allergic lung disorder caused by exposure to moldy hay. *See also* Hypersensitivity Pneumonitis.

Feathers Feathers are a common cause of respiratory allergies. Aged feathers, in contrast to fresh feathers, appear to be more allergenic, which suggests that the allergens responsible for the symptoms are products that degrade. The most common source of exposure to feathers at home is pillows. Other sources are mattresses, cushions, and upholstery. A patient who is allergic to one type of feather is usually allergic to other types. People sensitive to feathers do not experience allergic reactions from egg-containing vaccines unless they are also allergic to egg protein.

Food Allergy   Foods are intimately related to human existence, both physiologically and psychologically. For these reasons, it is understandable that people tend to associate food with a wide variety of manifestations of diseases. Foods may cause adverse reactions through a variety of mechanisms such as allergic reactions, contaminants that cause toxic reactions or infections, food intolerance, and psychological mechanisms. The term *food allergy* is frequently misused by both people and physicians in referring to a variety of symptoms ranging from true allergies to vague, common complaints such as fatigue, tension, low energy, and headaches. Loose application of the word *allergy* to food has rendered the term almost useless in describing allergies that may or may not be related to the intake of food. Unequivocal clinical symptoms produced by foods are uncommon; perhaps less than 1 percent of infants exhibit allergy to cow's milk, and this may be one of the more common examples. Although foods may be important in cases of infantile eczema, urticaria, or anaphylaxis, they are relatively unimportant in most cases of allergic conjunctivitis, rhinitis, and asthma.

Immunological reactions to foods are commonly divided into two groups, allergic (IgE) mediated and nonallergic mediated. The allergic mediated reaction is more common in children than in adults. Symptoms usually appear a few minutes to a few hours after ingestion of the food, and they may be manifested by hives, angioedema, rash, asthma, abdominal symptoms such as diarrhea, vomiting, or abdominal pain, as well as by other anaphylactic symptoms. In clearcut cases of food allergy, skin tests by the prick method are usually positive for the foods in question. In a recent study involving more than one hundred infants and children, the following foods were found to be important causes of symptoms: soybean, cow's milk, peanuts and other nuts, and eggs.

Nonallergic mediated reactions are reactions to foods that are mediated by other immunological mechanisms. Symptoms are malabsorption in the gastrointestinal tract, a disease of the intestines in which protein is lost; vomiting; and chronic diarrhea, among others. Respiratory symptoms such as pneumonia, cough, or asthma, and skin blemishes such as hives or angioedema may also appear. Symptoms occur several hours to a few days after the food is eaten, in contrast to a few minutes to a few hours in the case of allergic (IgE) reactions. This delay makes it more difficult to establish an association between the symptoms and the food taken. Cow's milk is the food most often responsible for such reactions; usually it causes primarily gastrointestinal and respiratory symptoms.

Table 2.2. Major Groups of Allergenic Foods

Cashew (Anacardiaceae)	Cashew, mango, pistachio
Cereal grasses (Gramineae)	Bamboo, barley, corn, oats, rice, rye, sugar cane, wheat
Citrus (Rutaceae)	Grapefruit, lemon, orange, tangerine
Cola nut (Sterculiaiceae)	Chocolate, cola nut
Goosefoot (Chenopodiaceae)	Beet, lamb's quarter, spinach
Legume (Leguminosae)	Beans, peas, soybean, peanut, lentil, licorice
Lily (Liliaceae)	Asparagus, garlic, onion, sarsaparilla
Mallow (Malvaceae)	Cottonseed, marshmallow, okra
Melon (Cucurbitaceae)	Cantaloupe, cucumber, pumpkin, squash, watermelon
Mustard (Cruciferae)	Broccoli, cabbage, horseradish, mustard
Nightshade (Solanaceae)	Eggplant, potato, tomato
Plum (Amygdalaceae)	Almond, apricot, cherry, peach, plum
Rose (Rosaceae)	Raspberry, strawberry
Sunflower (Compositae)	Artichoke, chicory, dandelion, lettuce, sunflower seed
Walnut (Juglandaceae)	Hickory nut, walnut, pecan

Fungi (Molds)   Fungi are plants that, unlike green plants, have no chlorophyll and must depend on plant or animal material for nourishment. About 100,000 species of fungi have been identified. Many species can be the cause of disease in humans, animals, and plants. Molds, however, may be beneficial by increasing in the decay of vegetation or as a source of antibiotics and enzymes.

The greatest number of fungi are produced by the soil. Temperature, humidity, and air circulation are some of the meteorological factors that determine fungal growth and distribution. In warm, humid climates, molds are present in large quantities almost all year round. They grow best at temperatures between 70 and 90 degrees Fahrenheit (21 and 32 degrees Celsius) and stop growing below 40 degrees Fahrenheit (4 degrees Celsius). Indoor molds are essentially similar to outdoor molds; their growth depends on the same factors that enable them to grow outdoors. The most common sites of mold growth are vegetable containers; house plants; furniture; refrigerator and air-conditioner drip trays; most organic substances such as wool, carpets, and wallpaper; and damp cellars and closets.

Molds reproduce by spores that, like pollen, are shed in large quantities into the air. Fungal spores are present in the air in concentrations that significantly exceed the concentration of pollen grains. Worldwide, cladosporium is probably the most widely distributed mold. Among the fungal classes, families of the *Fungi Imperfecti* class, such as cladosporium, alternaria, aspergillus, and penicillium, are known to produce allergic symptoms in humans. Information about the role of fungi spores in allergic diseases, however, has been limited to a few members of the *Fungi Imperfecti* class, and little is known about the role of other fungi classes such as mushrooms in causing allergic diseases. *See also* Molds.

Gamma Globulins   Gamma globulins are a restricted group of proteins obtained by the electrophoretic separation of serum proteins. Included are all the immunoglobulins that possess specific antibody activity against many foreign substances and are important in defense mechanisms against these substances. Commercial preparations of gamma globulins are available for treating patients with severe deficiencies in antibody production, as well as for treating those with certain diseases.

Gastroenteritis   Gastroenteritis is an inflammation of the stomach and intestines. It may at times result from an allergic reaction.

Genetic Markers   Genetic markers are inherited features that scientists are identifying and that may enable them to understand the inherited aspects of many normal and abnormal processes in the body; some markers for which tests exist can predict who is at high risk of inheriting or developing specific diseases.

Glues and Gums   Glues and gums can occasionally cause allergies. Chicle, gum arabic, acacia, and other vegetable gums have been reported as causing allergy by inhalation or ingestion. They are present in many common foods and medications.

Goosefoot and Careless Weed   The goosefoot and careless weed (Chemopodiaceae and Amaranthacae) families produce abundant pollen that is highly allergenic. These weeds are particularly im-

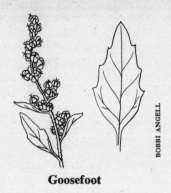

BOBBI ANGELL

Goosefoot

portant in the Great Plains and the Southwest. The most important member of the group is Russian thistle.

Grasses   Grasses are widely distributed and include more than 4,000 species. Most of the wild native grasses produce very little pollen, leaving few introduced species as the major source of pollen. In the South, grass pollen may be encountered during most of the year. In colder regions, the season extends from mid-May to the end of July. In the Northeast, the bulk of the grass pollen is derived from bluegrass, timothy, orchard, and redtop. Velvet grass and rye grass are common on the Pacific coast. Bermuda is a dominant lawn and field grass in the southern states. Recently, Bahia grass has also become an important source of grass pollen in the South. Grasses are the major cause of hay fever in the United States during the summer.

Hay Fever   Hay fever is a common name for nasal allergy. Its symptoms—attacks of sneezing, runny, stuffy nose, and itchy, watery eyes—occur within a few minutes to a few hours after exposure to inhaled allergens—usually pollen, spores from molds, house dust, or animal danders. The term *hay fever* is misleading, since these reactions are not usually produced by hay and are not accompanied by fever.
   See also Rhinitis.

Histamine   Histamine is a chemical released in the body by the interaction of an allergen and an antibody; it is believed to cause the swelling and itching that accompany allergic skin disorders and the symptoms of allergic rhinitis.

Histamine-Release Test   A histamine-release test is a method of measuring the amount of histamine released by certain cells in a sample of blood from an allergic patient when the cells are exposed to an allergen; the test is used to gain some idea of a patient's reactivity to specific substances. The test is currently used only in major research centers, and requires sophisticated equipment.

Hives   *See* Urticaria.

House Dust   House dust is a heterogeneous, firm gray powdery material that accumulates indoors. This category includes mold, pollen, animal danders, food particles, kapok, cotton linters, insects, and bacteria. Aggravation of respiratory symptoms by exposure to dust is common. Symptoms may be due to an irritant, or they may have an allergic basis. Allergy to dust is regarded by many allergists as one of the most common causes of perennial rhinitis. The allergenicity of house dust cannot be explained by the presence of pollen, molds, or animal danders. The identification of allergenic material in house dust has been the subject of many scientific investigations. Some researchers believe that the main allergen in house dust is degenerative cellulose. Although it is not known whether there is a specific allergen in house dust, there is no doubt that house dust contains allergens capable of producing symptoms in allergenic patients. These allergens play an important role in numerous cases of rhinitis and asthma.

Recently, several investigators have demonstrated that house dust mites (dermatophagoides) may be a primary source of house dust allergens. Mites are common contaminants of house dust; certain conditions such as high humidity and the presence of danders increase the number of mites. Available data suggests that mites are a major source of dust allergen, but that they are not the only causative agent in dust.

Hypergammaglobulinemia   When the level of gamma globulins in the blood increases, a person is said to have hypergammaglobulinemia. The condition may reflect a response to a chronic infection, or it may be part of a chronic inflammatory reaction associated with a number of diseases. Higher levels of gamma globulin may also be a compensatory mechanism in cases where there is less synthesis of albumin or an overproduction of an abnormal immunoglobulin called a paraprotein or myeloma protein.

Hypersensitivity   Hypersensitivity is a condition in which the immune system reacts to antigens that cause tissue damage and disease. This is in contrast to the normal beneficial effect of the immune response. Hypersensitivity reactions are usually divided into the following four main types:

Anaphylactic This type is mediated by allergic (IgE) antibodies. Hay fever, certain types of asthma, hives, some food and drug reactions, and systemic anaphylaxis are examples. *See also* Anaphylaxis.

Cytotoxic In this type of reaction, antibodies of the IgG and IgM classes react with antigens present in cell membranes. The antigen-antibody reaction activates the complement system, culminating in lysis (destruction) of the cell. An example of this type of reaction is the destruction of red blood cells that occurs as a result of an auto-immune reaction.

Immune-complex mediated This type of reaction results from deposits of antigen-antibody complexes in different tissues. The complement system is also involved. Examples of this type of reaction are serum sickness, some types of drug reactions, and certain renal diseases.

Delayed, or cell-mediated hypersensitivity Delayed hypersensitivity is a form of immune response characterized by a process of inflammation that reaches its maximum intensity twenty-four to forty-eight hours after exposure to the offending substance, or antigen. Common examples are the skin lesions associated with contact to poison ivy and metals and the reaction to numerous fungi, viruses, and transplanted organs. It is mediated by sensitized lymphocytes. *See also* Allergy.

Hypersensitivity Pneumonitis Hypersensitivity pneumonitis is an allergic disease of the lungs caused by inhaling various organic dusts. A person suffering from the disease shows symptoms similar to those of flu: fever, aching, and difficulty breathing. Hypersensitivity pneumonitis occurs four to six hours after inhalation of the dusts. Prolonged low-grade exposure to such dusts may result in more insidious illness characterized by gradual onset of shortness of breath at the time of exercise.

The exact immune mechanism responsible for the disease has not been established. Antigen-antibody reactions, as well as cell-mediated immune responses, are believed to be implicated as causes of the lung damage that results. Hypersensitivity pneumonitis has numerous causes (see Table 2.2). Although most of the recognized causes are found in the workplace, the disease may be related to a hobby or it may result from exposure to a variety of microorganisms that contaminate humidifiers and air-conditioner systems. General treatment consists of avoiding further exposure, and severe conditions are treated with corticosteroids (cortisone).

Table 2.3. Causes of Hypersensitivity Pneumonitis

DISEASE	EXPOSURE TO
Farmer's lung	Moldy hay and other fodder
Bagassosis	Moldy sugar cane
Mushroom worker's disease	Mushroom compost
Humidifier (ventilation) disease	Contaminated humidifying or ventilation systems
Malt worker's disease	Moldy malt
Sauna taker's disease	Contaminated appliance
Bird fancier's disease (pigeon breeders lung)	Droppings of pigeons, budgerigars (small Australian parrots), parrots, chicken hens, or turkeys
Maple bark stripper's disease	Moldy maple logs
Sequoiosis	Moldy redwood sawdust
Wood pulp worker's disease	Moldy logs
Pituitary snuff taker's disease	Desiccated pituitary
Suberosis	Moldy cork dust
Cheesewasher's disease	Cheese mold
Wheat weevil disease	Wheat flour
Furrier's lung	Hair dust
Coffee worker's lung	Coffee dust
Thatched roof (New Guinea) lung	Thatched roof dust
Vineyard sprayer's lung	Vineyards
Duck fever	Feathers
Miller's lung	Contaminated grain
Turkey handler's disease	Turkey products
Paprika slicer's lung	Moldy paprika pods

Hypoallergenic Agents   A hypoallergenic substance is one that is less likely to cause an allergenic reaction; according to the Food and Drug Administration, however, it has not been proved that any product is, indeed, hypoallergenic, despite claims by manufacturers to the contrary.

Hypogammaglobulinemia Hypogammaglobulinemia occurs when there is a decreased level of gamma globulin in the blood. It may be due to failure in the gamma globulin-producing cells (B lymphocytes) or to greater losses through the kidneys, the gastrointestinal tract, or skin. The disease may also be secondary to other diseases that damage the gamma globulin-producing cells.

Hyposensitization Hyposensitization is a method of treating allergies in which series of small doses of the substance that causes an allergy are administered in increasingly large concentrations, in the hope of increasing a person's immunity to the substance. The method is also known as densensitization or immunotherapy. *See also* immunotherapy.

Idiosyncratic Reaction *See* Reaction, Idiosyncratic.

Immune A condition in which an organism is protected against, or free from, the effects of allergy or infection, either by already having had the disease or by inoculation, is called an immune condition.

Immunoglobulins Immunoglobulin is one of a family of proteins to which antibodies belong.
Immunoglobulin A Abbreviated IgA, a class of globulins containing antibody activity found in such body secretions as saliva, tears, or intestinal and bronchial fluids. IgA serves as the first line of defense against organisms that invade the respiratory or gastrointestinal systems.
Immunoglobulin D Abbreviated IgD, a class of globulins containing antibody activity present in extremely low concentrations; its exact role is unknown.
Immunoglobulin E Abbreviated IgE, a class of globulins containing antibody activity normally present in extremely small quantities in humans but found in larger amounts in people with allergies and certain infections. Although its role in protection is not known, medical evidence indicates that IgE is solely responsible for classic allergy symptoms.
Immunoglobulin G Abbreviated IgG, the most abundant class of immunoglobulin containing antibody activity. The major serum against invading organisms immunoglobulin produced by the body.
Immunoglobulin M Abbreviated IgM, a class of globulins con-

taining antibody activity produced in early immune responses and effective as an initial defense against bacteria.

Immunotherapy   The form of treatment known as immunotherapy is also called desensitization, hyposensitization, or allergy shots. Immunotherapy is used in the treatment of allergic patients with respiratory symptoms, mainly of hay fever or asthma. In this form of treatment, injections of allergenic extract are given in gradually increasing amounts of allergenic extract over a period of months. The goal is to induce a degree of tolerance to the allergens and to bring about a decline in the symptoms and the medication requirements.

The mechanism involved is not entirely clear. Among the changes that occur in patients after immunotherapy are the development of blocking IgG antibodies (protective antibodies), a gradual decline in the level of allergic (IgE) antibodies against the offending substance, and a decrease in the patient's cell sensitivity for the release of histamine upon exposure to the allergen. Although no uniform schedule or dosage has been established for administering allergenic extracts, strong scientific evidence exists to support the belief that greater amounts of extract administered to a patient produce more satisfactory results than do smaller doses. The administration of very small doses of allergenic extract is popular among some specialists, but such treatment is not supported by adequate experimental studies. Currently, the main use of immunotherapy is in treating patients who are sensitive to inhaled allergens, mainly pollen, mold, and house dust. The administration of food extracts to patients highly sensitive to foods is contraindicated because of the chance of a severe anaphylactic reaction. Immunotherapy involving food extracts in patients with low sensitivity to food allergens has not been demonstrated as valid in well-designed clinical studies.

Ingestant Allergen   An ingestant allergen is a substance that causes an allergic reaction when eaten or swallowed—for example, eggs, milk, aspirin, or penicillin.

Inhalant Allergen   An inhalant allergen is one that enters the body through the respiratory system—for example, pollen, mold spores, or animal dander.

Inhalation Challenge   Inhalation challenge is a test used in the reproduction of allergic symptoms by breathing an offending substance, or allergen, into the nose or the bronchial tubes. The effect of doing this is then compared with that produced when a control substance, such as saline, is used. The inhalation challenge test is highly specific, but it has several limitations when used as a routine test in clinical practice. Not least among these limitations are the time involved (for the patient as well as the physician) and the cost. There is, however, a good correlation between the results obtained with the inhalation challenge test, using a major allergen, and skin tests with the prick method.

Insect Allergy The insects responsible for allergic reactions are almost exclusively in the class Hymenoptera. The most important are yellow jackets, hornets, wasps, honeybees, and fire ants. Allergy to insects may affect individuals who are either allergic (atopic) or non-allergic to common pollens and molds. Reactions may be local and are characterized by swelling, redness, and pain, or they may be systemic. Examples of systemic reactions are: generalized urticaria (hives); bronchospasm (asthma-like symptoms); throat swelling; and in some patients, low blood pressure. Severe systemic (anaphylactic) reactions may be fatal if not treated promptly. Anaphylactic reactions are mediated by allergic antibodies directed against components of the insect venom. Following the sting and penetration of the venom, the venom antigens react with the allergic antibodies present on the surface of mast cells and basophils. These antigen-antibody reactions initiate a series of intracellular events that culminate in the release of several active chemicals such as histamine. The action of these compounds on the various tissues is responsible for the symptoms of allergy in a person. The presence of significant amounts of allergic antibodies directed against insect venom can be demonstrated in an individual by skin tests or by a laboratory test, using the individual's serum; the test is known as a radioallergosorbent (RAST) test. *See* RAST.

In recent years the treatment of highly allergic patients has been improved significantly with the introduction of better allergenic materials for diagnosing and treating insect allergy. Today, it is recommended that patients with a clinical history of severe anaphylactic reactions to insect venom, and high levels of allergic antibodies, be treated by immunotherapy, starting with small doses of venom extract and increasing the dosage.

Following are the main characteristics of insects that cause allergic reactions:

Yellow Jackets Bands of yellow and black around the thorax and abdomen. The head is yellow and black. Yellow jackets are second only to hornets in aggressiveness and are frequently seen near garbage and picnic areas. Their nests are large and are usually

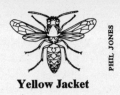

Yellow Jacket

located in the ground, often in tall grass between the walls of buildings or under stones.

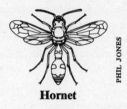

Hornet

Hornets Black body with white markings on the thorax and abdomen. The face, excluding the top of the head, is also white. Hornets may be difficult to distinguish from yellow jackets, since they often have yellow markings. Hornets' nests are large, gray, or brown and are located in tree branches, under the eaves of houses, or against a wall, usually more than four feet above the ground. Hornets are considered the most aggressive of the major stinging insects, sometimes attacking without apparent provocation.

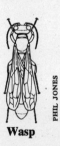

Wasp

Wasps Black or brown with yellow or white stripes and a fusiform (tapering toward each end) abdomen. The wasp can be distinguished from the yellow jacket and the hornet by its thin waist, which joins the abdomen and the thorax. Wasps are not as excitable as the other stinging insects; they usually sting only if touched or brushed while in flight around the nest. They build their nests in trees or around shelters such as the eaves of houses or porches. The nest is usually small and contains thirty to sixty insects.

Honeybee

Honeybees Easily recognized by their small, stocky, brown, yellow, or black bodies with a round abdomen. Probably the best-known insect, honeybees are found most frequently in artificial hives, but the colonies may be found in natural nests inside the trunks of trees, under floorboards, and in other enclosed areas. The stinger differs from that of the yellow jacket, wasp, or hornet, in that it cannot be used repeatedly (the stinging apparatus is severed from the body after the sting, the stinger is left in the skin, and the bee dies).

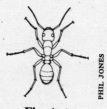

Fire Ant

Fire Ants Introduced from South America during the 1920s, fire ants are now well established in several Southern states. The venom of the fire ant differs from that of hymenoptera insects, in that it can produce severe local reactions or systemic anaphylactic reactions. The insect attacks by biting to secure itself, then inserts its stinging apparatus, which contains the venom. Highly sensitive patients with high levels of allergic antibodies against the venom of the fire ant are usually treated with immunotherapy.

Someone who is sensitive to insect bites should avoid:

1. Standing in the direct path of a flight of insects
2. Contact with a nest
3. Throwing objects at a nest
4. Mowing the lawn
5. Planting flowers
6. Trimming hedges or shrubs
7. Painting houses

8. Handling trash or garbage cans
9. Walking barefoot outdoors
10. Cooking or eating outdoors
11. Using scented preparations such as perfume, hairsprays, colognes, or deodorants
12. Wearing brightly colored clothing with flower patterns

Intrinsic Asthma   *See* Asthma, Intrinsic.

Iodism   Iodism is a group of symptoms that often accompany the chronic use of iodide drugs.

Kapok   Kapok is a vegetable fiber from the kapok tree. It was once widely used as stuffing for pillows, mattresses, sleeping bags, and cushions. Its allergenicity appears to be associated with aging of the fibers. In recent years, it has largely been replaced by synthetic materials.

Leukocytosis   Leukocytosis is a condition characterized by an increased number of white blood cells.

Leukotrienes   *See* Arachidonic Acid.

Lymphocyte   A lymphocyte is a white blood cell important in immunity; of the two major types (both types have several subclasses), T lymphocytes are processed in the thymus and are involved in cell-mediated immunity, and B lymphocytes are derived from the bone marrow and are precursors of plasma cells, which produce antibody.

Macrophage   A macrophage is a scavenger white blood cell that plays a role in destroying invading bacteria and other foreign material. It also plays a major role in the immune response by processing or handling antigens and as an effector cell in delayed hypersensitivity.

Mast Cell   A mast cell is a type of tissue cell containing the chemical mediators responsible for the symptoms of allergy; when allergens attach to IgE antibodies lying on the surface of these cells, a signal is sent, causing them to release the chemical mediators of allergy.

Mediator   A mediator is a chemical substance that attracts or activates other parts of the immune system—for example, histamine.

Medic Alert Bracelet   An identification bracelet is provided to a person who may have a severe allergy such as an insect sting reaction by Medic Alert, a nonprofit organization on call twenty-four hours a day; the address is P. O. Box 1009, Turlock, CA 95380.

Methylxanthine   *See* Bronchodilator.

Mixed Asthma   *See* Asthma, Mixed.

Molds (Fungi)   *Mold* is a general term for a group of parasitic, microscopic plants without stems, roots, or leaves and composed of a vegetative threadlike element (hyphae) and a reproductive element (spores). *See also* Fungi.

Mucolytic   A substance used to thin secretions.

Mucus   Mucus is a glutinous secretion of the mucous membranes; it is produced by glands to protect and moisten the membranes.

Nasal Polyps   Nasal polyps are round, small, smooth, soft masses—single or multiple—that form in the sinus or nasal cavities. They can occur in patients with severe allergies, or they may appear as a result of chronic inflammation in patients with vasomotor rhinitis. In some patients, polyps occur without a discernible cause. Removal of the polyps by surgery may be necessary, especially when they obstruct the nasal passages; but in some cases, polyps can be treated with cortisone.

Orris Root   A powdered product made from plants of the orris family, orris root was once widely used as a powder base in cosmetics. Because of the number of people with allergic reactions to the root, however, it has been virtually abandoned.

Otitis Media (Serous)   Otitis media is an inflammation of the middle ear, frequently seen in young children. It may also be found in children with allergic symptoms and may be complicated by secondary bacterial infections. In children with severe allergies, control of the allergic problem is often associated with improvement of the otitis media. If fluid accumulates behind the tympanic membrane (ear drum), hearing may be affected.

Patch Test   Patch tests are used to identify substances responsible for contact allergy. The test consists of applying a small amount of a suspected substance to the skin. The area is then covered with tape and left for forty-eight hours. If a small area where the substance was applied swells and turns red, the test result is said to be positive.

Penicillium   Penicillium are fungi that belong to the class Fungi Imperfecti. These fungi are a common cause of rot in storage grain and in fruits and vegetables; they are also often found in houses, especially in their basements. Penicillium can produce allergic symptoms such as hay fever and asthma in allergic patients. *See also* Fungi; Molds.

Pericarditis   Pericarditis is an inflammation of the membrane covering the heart.

Pituitary Gland   The pituitary gland is a small oval endocrine gland at the base of the brain; it secretes several hormones, one of which regulates the secretion of cortisone by the adrenal gland. *See also* cortisone.

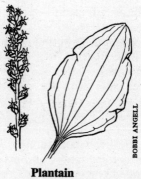

Plantain

Plantain Family   Of the plantain family (Plantaginaceae), English plantain is the best-known species. It is wind-pollinated and may cause hay fever during the summer. Pollination occurs from June to August.

Pneumonia, Allergic   Allergic pneumonia is an inflammation of the lungs resulting directly from an allergy, usually to some type of organic dust. *See also* Hypersensitivity Pneumonitis.

Pneumonitis, Hypersensitivity   *See* Hypersensitivity Pneumonitis.

Pollen   Pollen contains the male fertilizing elements of a plant and is microscopic in size. Pollen grains are spheroid, ovoid, or ellipsoid in shape and may have a smooth, reticulated, spiculated, or sculptured surface. These surface characteristics are used for identifying pollen grains in atmospheric surveys. The problems that confront the pollen grain in accomplishing its function (pollination) are those of reaching the pistil of another flower. The more primitive method of pollination is the dispersion of pollen grains by the wind. This method is not efficient and must be compensated for by the liberation of large amounts of pollen. Wind-pollinated plants are responsible for the majority of cases of allergic rhinitis, or hay fever. The other method of plant pollination is by insects. Wind-pollinated flowers can be distinguished from insect-pollinated flowers by the lack of qualities attractive to insects, such as color, perfume, and nectar. In general, the flowers important in the production of allergic symptoms are not the beautiful, conspicuous flowers, which are insect-pollinated, but those that share most pollen and are dull and unattractive. Each climatic area has its own particular group of hay-fever plants. The pollen season in most localities can be conveniently divided into three distinct seasons—spring, early summer, and late summer and fall.

Spring coincides with the flowering of such trees as elm, juniper, oak, birch, and willow. Because this season is short, it is less important than the other two.

Early summer coincides with the pollination of grasses, which are of primary importance in the production of hay fever. The duration of this season varies with the latitude and is longer in southern zones.

The season that includes late summer and fall corresponds to the flowering of the ragweed family and extends from mid-August to early October. Ragweed is considered the most important hay-fever-producing plant in the United States.

Polymyositis   Polymyositis is a painful inflammation of several muscles at once; it may occur in conjunction with presumably autoimmune diseases or in some cancer patients.

Prick Test   *See* Scratch Test.

Prostaglandins   *See* Arachidonic Acid.

Provocative Testing   *See* Challenge Test.

Psychogenic Disorder   A psychogenic disorder is one originating in the mind or in mental conflict.

RAGWEED DENSITY IN THE UNITED STATES

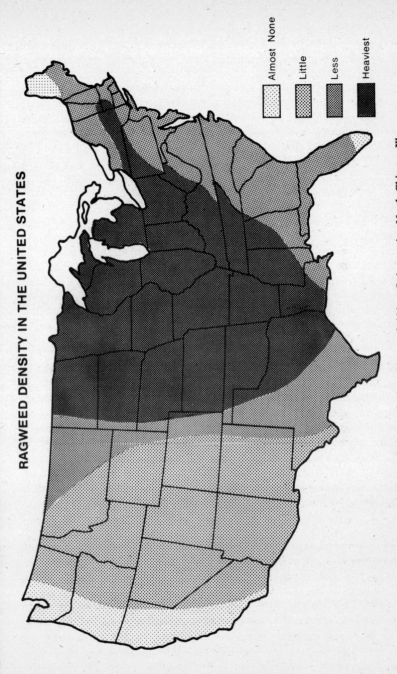

Almost None

Little

Less

Heaviest

Map provided through the courtesy of Abbott Laboratories, North Chicago, Ill.

Psychosomatic Disorder A psychosomatic disorder is one in which nonorganic or mental processes influence or directly cause an organic disease.

Pyrethrum Pyrethrum is prepared from the flower of the pyrethrum plant, a member of the ragweed family, and is widely used as an insecticide. It may act as an irritant or as a specific allergen. People who are allergic to ragweed may experience allergic symptoms when exposed to pyrethrum.

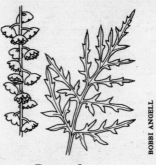

Ragweed

Ragweed Ragweed, a plant belonging to the family Compositae, is the major cause of hay fever in the United States. The ragweed (Compositae) family is large, with approximately 15,000 species. Although the number of wind-pollinated species is relatively low, they produce and release a tremendous amount of pollen. Members of the ragweed genus *Ambrosia* are plentiful over much of North America, growing as weeds in vacant lots, on farmland, and in cities and along the road. Ragweed plants are short-day plants that are brought into flower by the waning days of late summer. Ragweed-induced hay fever begins earlier in the northern latitudes than in the southern latitudes and usually extends to October. Because of the amount of agricultural land and the pattern of air movement across North America, few areas of the United States are free of ragweed. The areas with little ragweed are those forested with northern conifers, southern Florida, and most of the Southwest and Pacific coast.

RAST The RAST (for *radioallergosorbent test*) is used to detect and measure allergic antibodies against an antigen in a person's serum. It is more specific than skin tests but is less sensitive and more expensive. Currently it is being used in certain patients for whom skin tests are technically difficult, such as those with severe skin diseases and young children or infants.

Reaction, Anaphylactic An anaphylactic reaction is a state of shock caused by a severe allergic reaction, which results in sudden collapse and, occasionally, in death.

Reaction, Idiosyncratic An idiosyncratic reaction is similar to systemic allergic reaction, but in this type, allergic mechanisms cannot be demonstrated.

Reagin *Reagin* is a term used to describe allergic antibodies of the IgE type.

Rebound Phenomenon The rebound phenomenon is an allergy condition in which prolonged use of a drug or drugs (such as nasal vasoconstrictor sprays for hay fever treatment) creates a need for more and more of the drug(s), while the desired effect steadily decreases.

Receptors Receptors are sites on cell surfaces where drugs and other chemicals attach, enter, or activate.

Rejection Rejection is the destruction of transplanted foreign tissues or cells by hypersensitivity reactions of the recipient; also called a graft rejection. There are several types of graft, depending on the species involved, and several patterns of graft rejection.

Rheumatoid Arthritis Rheumatoid arthritis is a disease characterized by chronic inflammation of the joints. It may also affect other organs and tissues of the body. Immunological factors are important in the origination and development of the disease. A specific antibody against denatured, or altered, gamma globulins—called rheumatoid factor— is often found in the serum of patients with rheumatoid arthritis.

Rhinitis Rhinitis is a disease of the nasal passages that is characterized by attacks of sneezing, increased nasal secretion, and stuffy nose (caused by swelling of the nasal mucosa). The symptoms may result from an allergic reaction, or they may be due to a nonspecific hyperactivity of the nasal mucosa (vasomotor rhinitis) in response to environmental irritants.
See also Allergic Rhinitis; Hay Fever.

Rhinitis Medicamentosa Rhinitis medicamentosa is a type of rhinitis that is induced by frequent and prolonged use of decongestant nasal drops and sprays. The nasal passages become red, boggy, or pale gray and edematous, and the inflamed membranes are indistinguishable from other forms of chronic inflammation of the nose, due to overuse of topical nasal decongestants.

Rhinitis, Perennial Allergic   Perennial allergic rhinitis is year-round hay fever.

Rinkel Desensitization   Rinkel desensitization is an unproven and controversial method of allergy desensitization involving "end point" titration skin testing. In this technique the amount of allergen given during desensitization is based on quantitative skin testing. A recent controlled double-blind study performed by highly qualified allergists at the Johns Hopkins Medical School has shown this method of treatment to be ineffective, in that it was no better than placebo (an inactive substance used in well-controlled clinical trials) in treating allergic rhinitis.

Scratch Test   A scratch test is an allergy skin test in which the allergen is applied directly to small scratches or needle pricks made in the skin.
   See also Prick Test.

Seed Allergens   Vegetable seeds contain proteins that can cause allergic reactions. The more potent allergens are present in cottonseed, castor beans, and flaxseed. A person may be exposed to these seeds by inhalation or ingestion. In the case of the castor bean, exposure by inhalation is usually restricted to workers handling the beans. Cotton linters attach to the seeds after processing and are a primary source of trouble from stuffed toys, mattresses, and furniture. Sources of inhaled flaxseed allergens are animal feed, lotions, and fertilizers.

Sensitize   *Sensitize* is synonymous with *immunize;* to administer or expose to an antigen provoking an immune response so that, upon later exposure to that antigen, a more vigorous secondary response will occur. An individual can be immune (for example, protected against the effects of an infectious agent or antigen) and sensitized to the antigen (for example, demonstrate a positive tuberculin reaction) at the same time.
   See also Immune.

Serotonin   Serotonin is a body chemical that causes a variety of effects such as contraction of smooth muscle; it plays a role in anaphylactic reactions in several species of animals, but its role in allergic reactions in humans is not yet known.

Serum Serum is the yellow liquid part of the blood that remains after cells and fibrin have been removed.

Serum Sickness Serum sickness was originally described as an allergic illness that occurs six to eight days after administration of large amounts of an animal antiserum. The patient develops fever; skin lesions, particularly urticaria (hives); pain and swelling in the joints; and swelling in the lymph nodes. Symptoms may be mild, lasting only a few days, or they may be severe, involving numerous organs, including the heart and kidneys. The mechanism responsible for serum sickness consists of deposits of antigen-antibody complexes (animal serum protein being the antigen, combined with human antibodies) in various organs and tissues. These antigen-antibody complexes activate the complement system and subsequently induce the process of inflammation responsible for the tissue damage and symptoms.

In the past, horse antitoxin, or antiserum (that is, a foreign, animal serum protein) was widely used in treating bacterial infection, but its use was often complicated by serum sickness. Recently, the primary use of horse serum has been against powerful toxins such as snake and spider venom and as a preparation of antilymphocyte serum used in organ transplants. Both drugs and serums can cause serum sickness, with penicillin currently the most frequent cause. Treatment is symptomatic; the choice of therapy depends on the clinical symptoms. Mild cases may require rest and the administration of such anti-inflammatory drugs as aspirin and antihistamines over a period of a few days. More severe cases may require the administration of a short course of corticosteroids such as prednisone. In the long run, however, the best way to prevent serum sickness is to avoid using animal serum and any drug unless the drug is absolutely necessary.

Shock Organ A shock organ is the tissue or organ in which an allergic reaction occurs.

Skin Test Skin tests are a method of testing for allergic antibodies. A test consists of introducing small amounts of the suspected substance, or allergen, into the skin and noting the development of a positive reaction (which consists of a wheal, swelling, or flare in the surrounding area of redness). The results are read fifteen to twenty minutes after application of the allergen. The three main skin tests used are:

Scratch Test In this method, a small drop of the allergen is applied over an area of the skin where a superficial scratch has been made. This allows the allergen to penetrate the top layer of skin.

Prick Method Here, the skin in pricked with a needle where a drop of allergen has already been placed.

Intradermal Method This method consists of injecting small amounts of an allergen into the superficial layers of the skin.

Interpreting the clinical significance of skin tests requires skillful correlation of the test results with the patient's clinical history. Positive tests indicate the presence of allergic antibodies and are not necessarily correlated with clinical symptoms.
See also prick test; scratch test.

Slow-Reacting Substance of Anaphylaxis Abbreviated SRS-A, this substance is a chemical that is released during an allergic reaction. It is a powerful bronchial constrictor and probably plays an important role in the bronchospasm associated with asthma.

Specificity Specificity is the characteristic of antibodies and white blood cells that enables them to recognize and interact only with the specific antigen they were produced to combat.

Spirometer A spirometer is a device that measures the amount of air inhaled and exhaled; it is used by physicians to measure the amount of airway obstruction in patients with asthma.

Spores Spores are the reproductive cells of certain plants and organisms. Inhaled fungal spores are frequently the cause of allergic symptoms such as rhinitis and asthma. *See also* allergens; fungi; molds.

Sputum In respiratory diseases, sputum is the discharge from air passages; it contains mucus and sometimes pus, bacteria, and other matter.

Status Asthmaticus Status asthmaticus is a severe asthma attack that does not respond to conventional therapy. It necessitates hospitalization and more vigorous treatment.

Steroid   *See* Cortisone.

Subcutaneous   *Subcutaneous* is an adjective meaning "under the skin."

Systemic Lupus Erythematosus   Systemic lupus erythematosus, abbreviated SLE, is an autoallergic disease. It frequently affects young women and may involve many different organs. In more serious cases, the kidneys and brain are often involved. Patients with SLE exhibit a variety of antibodies, which are directed against nuclear components of their cells. Detection of these antibodies (antinuclear antibodies) in the serum is helpful in diagnosis. The cause of SLE is unknown, but immunological factors acting on a suitable genetic background are believed important. There appears to be an important loss of immune regulatory function with decrease in suppressor T cell activity in SLE.

T Cells   T cells are white blood cells produced by the bone marrow and processed by the thymus. Also called T lymphocytes, these cells are responsible for cellular immunity and delayed hypersensitivity. There are many known subtypes of T cells, with varying functions (for example, "killer," "helper," "suppressor") that either enhance or suppress immune responses.

Thromboxane   *See* Arachidonic Acid.

Tobacco Sensitivity   Many people suffering from rhinitis and asthma experience heightened symptoms when exposed to tobacco smoke. Other clinical conditions have been associated with putative allergy to tobacco smoke, including various forms of dermatitis, cardio-vascular disturbances, gastrointestinal symptoms, and headaches. Whether these symptoms are caused by an allergic reaction to smoke allergens or to an irritative effect of smoke has yet to be resolved. Some investigations have demonstrated the presence of positive skin tests to tobacco-leaf extracts, as well as clinical improvement following immunotherapy in selected patients. Other studies, however, have failed to confirm these results. Most published studies have used tobacco-leaf extract rather than smoke extract and have lacked good experimental design and proper controls. The phrase *allergy to cigarette smoke* has become a highly emotional issue and is used loosely by the general public. At the present time, specific allergens in cigarette smoke have not been identified conclusively. In view of the irritative effect of cigarette smoke on the respiratory tract, and the sensitivity reported in many patients with respiratory allergies, such patients should avoid smoking and smoke should be eliminated as nearly as possible from home and work environments.

Toxin   A toxin is poison produced by a living organism.

Tree Pollen   Trees, important in respiratory allergy, are divided into the following families: conifers (Pinaceae); maple (Aceraceae); birch (Betulaseae); elm (Ulmaceae); willow and poplar (Salicaceae); walnut and hickory (Juglandaceae); and oak (Fagaceae). Tree pollen is an important cause of spring hay fever symptoms.

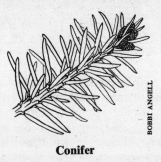

BOBBI ANGELL

Conifer

The conifer family includes pine, cedar, juniper, and black hemlock, among others. Conifers are the most common trees in Canadian forests, in the pinelands of the American Southeast and at lower elevations of the Rocky Mountains. Pollen production is substantial. Despite the widespread belief that pine pollen has strong allergenic qualities, the pollen is of little importance in respiratory allergy.

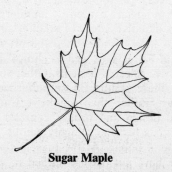

Sugar Maple

The maple family is widely distributed throughout the United States. Most maples are better suited for insect pollination, but they also depend partly on the wind. Pollination occurs in March and April and may produce symptoms common to early spring.

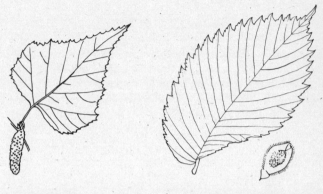

Gray Birch   **American Elm**

Birch, ironwood, alder, and hazelnut are members of the birch family. Abundant throughout the American Northeast, they produce significant amounts of pollen and are a major cause of hay fever in the early spring.

Distributed virtually throughout the United States, elms are among the earliest flowering trees in the spring. The elm produces large amounts of pollen, which is a cause of hay fever. In recent years the number of elms has decreased sharply because of a widespread fungus infection.

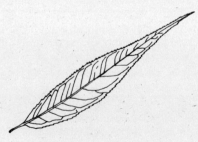

Babylon Weeping Willow

Willows are partially adapted to insect pollination, which occurs during March, April, and May. Poplars shed large amounts of pollen, are wind-pollinated, and cause hay fever in the early spring.

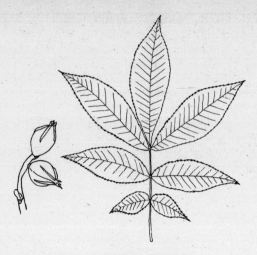

Bitternut Hickory

The walnut-hickory family includes walnut, hickory, and pecan trees. These species are common in the eastern, southern, and central states of the United States. The trees pollinate during the late spring and are a major cause of hay fever.

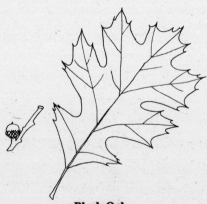

Black Oak

The oak family is made up primarily of oaks and beeches. These trees are widely distributed over the United States and produce an abundant amount of pollen, which is a major cause of hay fever during April and May.

Urticaria Urticaria, or hives, is a common skin condition that is probably familiar to everyone. It is a skin rash characterized by areas of localized swelling, usually very itchy and red, and occurring in various parts of the body. It usually lasts only a few hours and involves only the superficial areas of the skin. Urticaria has either an immunological or a nonimmunological cause.

Angioedema is a similar condition, but involves the subcutaneous tissue. It ordinarily does not itch and is a more generalized swelling.

See also Angioedema; Hives.

Vaccination Vaccination is the administration of specific weakened or killed antigens to stimulate the immune system so that the body will be protected against further exposure to the antigen.

Vasculitis Vasculitis is an inflammation of the blood vessels. There are several types of the disease; they are classified according to the size of the vessels, the organ or organs involved, and the cause. The existence of an immunological mechanism of the immune-complex type has been demonstrated in some cases of vasculitis.

Venoms *See* Insect Allergy.

Wheezing Wheezing is difficult, noisy breathing common in asthma sufferers.

Wool Wool fibers can irritate the skin or cause allergy by inhalation or contact. Such fibers are more common in atopic dermatitis than in rhinitis or asthma.

Yeasts Yeasts are species of fungi that grow as single cells. They may be prominent in the air during the fall months and during rainy weather. They may also contaminate cold steam vaporizers and aggravate asthma when devices of this type are not kept clean.

See also Fungi; Molds.

CHAPTER 3

Allergy Emergencies
and How to Cope with Them
by Harold S. Novey, M.D.

An emergency is an unforeseen condition, or set of circumstances, that requires prompt action. A true medical emergency is usually one in which the patient's life is threatened and the patient needs immediate medical attention. This definition implies that the medical condition is of very recent onset or that it is perhaps part of a chronic illness that has suddenly become more severe. Because it is sometimes difficult for either the patient or the physician to know whether the illness is immediately life-threatening, any similar condition that resulted in death should be considered life-threatening. This chapter deals mainly with such emergencies, as well as with serious but nonfatal, acute conditions.

Allergic emergencies are those associated with the classic allergy diseases asthma, hay fever, hives, and eczema, as well as allergic reactions to foreign matter, whether the matter is ingested, injected, inhaled, or absorbed by the skin. Although allergic diseases usually involve an immunological mechanism, some conditions closely resemble an allergic condition in which immunological causes may not have been demonstrated. These will also be discussed when appropriate.

Causes

Foreign substances are those that are not a natural, integral part of the body, that cause allergic reactions resulting in emergencies, or that produce fairly severe reactions. They are generally not dangerous—that is, they are not poisons, pathogenic organisms (such as viruses or bacteria), or radiation. These foreign, generally innocuous, substances are called, collectively, allergens. They may be inhaled, ingested, injected, or absorbed by the skin. They usually contain proteins that are medium-sized in molecular weight. Almost invariably, prior contact with either the identical agent or a closely related agent must occur before the allergic reaction is triggered.

Allergens that cause allergic reactions may be classified according to their sources, and are found in Table 3.1. Some of the drugs listed—for example, aspirin and the dyes used in x-ray studies—are not, strictly speaking, allergens, since a true immunological mechanism has not been found. The drugs are included both for traditional reasons and because they so closely reproduce reactions to true allergens.

Table 3.1. Causes of Allergic Reactions

ALLERGENS	EXAMPLES
Ingestants	
Foods	Shellfish, nuts, eggs, milk
Drugs	Penicillin, sulfa, aspirin
Inhalants	
Pollen	Airborne from certain grasses, weeds, trees containing house dust, animal danders, feathers, mold spores, insect parts
Industrial products	Isocyanates from polyurethane, formaldehydes, insecticides containing pyrethrums
Injectants	
Drugs	Penicillin, local anesthetics, some vaccines and hormones, radiopaque dyes used in x-ray studies, allergy extracts
Venom	Bees, yellow jackets, wasps, hornets, fire ants (hymenoptera)
Skin Contact	
Plants	Poison ivy, oak, sumac, primrose
Chemicals	Nickel-plated jewelry, cosmetics, perfumes
Medication	Antibiotic and antihistamine creams, suntan lotions

Symptoms, Diagnoses, and Variant Diagnoses

Emergencies

Anaphylaxis   Anaphylaxis is a sudden condition resembling shock that follows within minutes an allergic reaction to a foregn substance. It is potentially the most immediately life-threatening allergy emergency. If the allergen is ingested, as is the case with food or medication, the first symptom may be numbness or tingling in the mouth. This sensation may occur even before the food is completely chewed and swallowed, or it may begin within fifteen minutes after swallowing. The tongue swells, and the throat, or windpipe, feels constricted (from the ensuing edema, or swelling, of the soft tissues). In more severe reactions, the skin, cardiovascular, pulmonary, and gastrointestinal systems can, in rapid sequence, be affected. Hives, rapid heartbeat, lightheadedness, wheezing, nausea, and vomiting can be expected.

If the allergen is injected, either by the stinger of an insect or by a physician's needle, a red swelling at the site is likely to be the first sign. Then, except for a numbness and tingling in the mouth, symptoms similar to those when allergen is ingested may occur. The original site of contact with the allergen is thus involved initially, only to be followed rapidly by general symptoms. Fortunately, spontaneous recovery is the rule; a person recovers within thirty minutes to several hours, and the recovery is nearly always complete. In rare cases, the patient may faint from abnormally low blood pressure, experience seizures, or suffer cardiac damage.

Fatal anaphylaxis is rare. A Canadian study has uncovered seven such deaths per year in a population of 6 million. Although penicillin causes some reaction in about 10 percent of the people injected, the death rate is believed to be 1 in 7.5 million injections. Stinging insects inflict large, local (or nonfatal) anaphylactic reactions in slightly less than 1 percent of people stung. The death rate is about 1 per 3.5 million persons per year. In studies called urograms, radiologists and urologists inject radiocontrast dyes to better visualize the kidneys; it has been estimated that one death has occurred for every 116,000 such examinations. Reaction to an injected dye is called an anaphylactoid reaction. This type of reaction is similar to that of anaphylaxis, although no immunological basis has been discovered. X-ray dyes can release histamine and other chemical agents from cells in the body. For reasons that are poorly understood, in some people these drugs have an exaggerated capacity to act.

Why some people have these reactions and others do not has been attributed to a combination of the degree and type of exposure to the provoking agent, and to the immune system. Some individuals have inherited hyper-responding immune systems that produce more immunoglobulin E, as well as other antibodies. Repeated contact with small amounts of the allergen may have produced greater sensitization. Injections are more likely to cause general reactions than oral or skin contact. Death is more likely in people over forty or in those with chronic, severe health problems.

Variant Diagnosis Sometimes a person reacts to an injection by fainting. Before doing so, the individual becomes pale, light-headed, and possibly nauseous. Although the person may not suffer from hives or any respiratory difficulty, the pulse is apt to be slow. The individual revives after lying down. The cause is a nervous reaction (in medical terms, a vasovagal reaction) transmitted via the vagus nerve to the heart and blood vessels.

Table 3.2.   Allergic Reactions: Symptoms and Diagnoses

SYMPTOM	MEDICAL CONDITION
Difficulty breathing Shortness of breath	
Nose blocked	Hay fever, allergic rhinitis, nasal polyps
Throat blocked	Laryngeal edema—may be involved in anaphylaxis
Chest blocked	Asthma, anaphylaxis
Cough	Asthma, allergic rhinitis with postnasal drainage
Itching	
Skin	Eczema or atopic dermatitis, urticaria (hives), contact dermatitis
Nose and throat	Allergic rhinitis
Eyes	Allergic rhinitis and conjunctivitis
Swelling (edema)	
Parts of face and mouth, palms of hands, soles of feet	Angioedema—may occur alone or with anaphylaxis and serum sickness
Throat	Angioedema—may be involved in anaphylaxis and laryngeal edema
Eyes	Hay fever, allergic conjunctivitis, contact dermatitis
Skin	Hives
Pain	
Eyes	Allergic conjunctivitis
Ears	Allergic rhinitis with aerotitis or serous otitis media

Allergic Reactions: Symptoms and Diagnoses (cont.)

SYMPTOM	MEDICAL CONDITION
Throat	Allergic rhinitis with postnasal drainage; mouth breathing with nasal obstruction
Chest	Asthma attack and such complications as rib fracture from coughing; collapsed lung
Neck	More swelling than pain—escaped air under skin, called subcutaneous emphysema; over-use of accessory muscles of breathing with asthma
Abdomen	Asthma attack with overuse of abdominal muscles

Shortness of Breath and Other Breathing Problems Two conditions constitute an emergency in this category—laryngeal edema and asthma. Swelling of the windpipe, or laryngeal edema, is the most immediately life-threatening. The victim literally feels a lump in the throat, followed by a sensation of constriction and difficulty absorbing air, and produces a high-pitched, crowing sound. In other areas of the body, this swelling may be accompanied by hives or edema, or, as mentioned, it may be a manifestation of anaphylaxis. Such drugs as penicillin and its derivatives, and such foods as nuts and shellfish, are among the more common allergic causes. Insect stings, especially on the neck or face, may also be responsible.

Variant Diagnosis Anything that can block the windpipe can cause similar symptoms. This includes foreign bodies that enter the respiratory tract instead of the esophagus, infections that cause inflammation in the throat or the larynx, and tumors in these areas.

An asthma attack that is not relieved eventually becomes an emergency. A person with asthma cannot circulate air normally through the bronchial tubes. As these tubes become more constricted—due to contraction of their interlacing muscle, edema of their inner lining, or excess local production of mucus, among other factors—the asthma victim works harder and harder to breathe. The initial wheezing becomes louder, exhalation lasts longer, air is trapped inside, and the chest wall expands. The patient is forced to sit up with shoulders hunched forward. It becomes difficult to cough up the thickened mucus, and breathing becomes more and more labored. The symptoms of a serious asthma attack are:

1. An attack that does not improve after several hours have passed.
2. Wheezing that becomes louder and then stops, despite extremely labored breathing.
3. Increasing fatigue and weakness.
4. Pulse rate greater than 160 beats per minute in children under six, greater than 140 in others; or irregular rhythm.
5. Bulging of the neck muscles, an expanded chest cage, and deepening of the notch over the breastbone.

Fever is not a prominent factor in any of the emergency situations described thus far. If the asthma is complicated by an infection, the temperature usually exceeds 100° F (39° C).

Asthma also may be provoked by a viral respiratory infection such as influenza, in which case the patient suffers from both conditions. Asthma may also lead to pneumonia, a condition that may arise in a lung deprived of its normal oxygen supply by bronchial tubes obstructed by mucous plugs. In some cases, a relatively common airborne fungus spore grows in the air passages. An allergic reaction to the fungus produces inflammation that, in turn, causes a febrile bronchitis, or pneumonia. In medicine, this fungus is called aspergillus, and the complication, allergic bronchopulmonary aspergillosis.

If coughing is violent and prolonged, the opposing forces of chest muscles and rib muscles can cause a rib to fracture. Usually the rib does not break sufficiently to puncture the lungs, but the fractured rib can cause sharp chest pain. Coughing can also rupture air sacs in the lungs. The escaping air moves upward under the heart lining and the lung tissues. Trapped air causes a dull pain in the chest, or a sharp pain if part of a lung collapses under the pressure of trapped air (a condition known as pneumothorax). Often the air simply rises under the linings of the bronchial tubes to the trachea and stops in spaces beneath the soft neck tissues. The neck area will bulge and feel like crinkling paper to the touch (subcutaneous emphysema). This outcome—in reality, a safety mechanism—will be resolved and thereafter need not be considered a danger.

Variant Diagnosis Wheezing may also result from foreign objects or tumors in the bronchial tubes; infections in the tubes, called infectious bronchitis; chemical irritants entering the tubes, such as smoke, lyes, noxious gases; or fluid entering the tubes. Fluid may enter the lungs when a person is drowning, or it may originate internally because of damage to the blood vessels of the lungs. Prominent causes are congestive heart failure or pulmonary edema due to a failing heart, long-diseased lung tissue, and drugs such as heroin.

Skin Inflamation   The occasional skin reaction to a drug or plant, the last in this group of allergy emergencies, can become so extensive that it poses a real danger. Poison ivy or oak may produce such a skin reaction. The skin may blister. Intact skin protects against bacteria and allows the exchange of salts and water needed to prevent the body from overheating. If enough skin is involved, the victim risks complications from the partial loss of skin. If damage to the skin is extensive enough, fever, chills, skin abscesses, and blood-borne infections may occur.

The skin inflammation (dermatitis) that results from contact with poison ivy, cosmetics, metals, or chemicals is called, appropriately, contact dermatitis; antibodies are not involved. Cells called lympho-cytes become sensitized to the chemicals and, upon reexposure to the chemicals, enter the skin in an effort to remove the invading material. In the ensuing effort, the lymphocytes call in helper cells—macro-phages. Macrophages, literally "big eaters," may damage normal tissue in the process of clearing up the invaders. It generally takes about forty-eight hours after the chemical enters and the cells re-spond for skin damage to be visible.

An even more severe dermatitis may result—not from external contact this time, but from drugs taken internally. Some of the earlier, long-acting sulfa preparations were responsible for such severe blistering that large areas of the skin were shed, a condition physicians call exfoliative dermatitis. Today, few of the drugs com-monly used cause such reactions. It is always possible, however, that a new drug will be approved before an adverse reaction is discovered.

Severe anaphylaxis, unremitting asthma, acute edema of the larynx, and extensive contact (or exfoliative) dermatitis must all be considered true emergencies. Emergencies, though, may also arise from the side effects of the drugs used to treat these and other allergic diseases. Serious side effects are usually due to a relative over-dose of a drug. The overdose may be caused not only by receiving or taking more than the usually prescribed amount but because of the body's metabolism of the particular drug or because the excretion is slower than normal. The end result is an accumulation of high or toxic levels of the drug or drugs. Among antiallergy drugs, the bronchodilators used to treat asthma cause the bulk of serious side effects. (A list of undesirable reactions appears in Table 3.3.)

Table 3.3.   Acute Side Effects of Drugs Used in Allergy Treatment

DRUG GROUP	USES	SIDE EFFECTS
Aminophylline, theophylline	Bronchodilator— for asthma	Headache, nausea, vomiting, abdominal pain, rectal bleeding, drop in blood pressure, rapid or irregular heartbeat
Epinephrine, ephedrine, related adrenergics	Bronchodilator— for asthma, anaphylaxis, hives, angioedema	Headache, tremor, rapid or irregular heartbeat, rise in blood pressure, urinary retention in men
Steroids	Asthma; skin reactions	Hallucinations and delusions resembling psychosis, bleeding ulcer

Nonemergency Allergic Reactions

The conditions described below are more annoying than danger-ous. Familiarity with their symptoms and causes should alleviate alarm and lead to proper treatment.

Difficulty Breathing   Blockage of the nasal passages may result from congested nasal tissues caused by hay fever or allergic rhinitis. Other symptoms may be sneezing and watery blood-flecked nasal discharge from the nose or in the back of the throat or both. Throat tickle may provoke cough, and mild asthma may occur. These symptoms will not lead to total impairment of breathing, since breathing through the mouth can substitute for nasal obstruction. Nasal blockage may also result from polyps—nonmalignant growths of sinus and nasal tissue filled with fluid. If the blockage persists unabated for several days, both loss of smell and nasal and sinus infections may result.

Variant Diagnosis   Not all nasal symptoms are those of allergies. Simple colds or virus infections may simulate allergic disease. These can be distinguished by the presence of fever, general aching, and yellow or greenish nasal discharge. Usually an infection lasts about two weeks, whereas an allergic condition comes and goes over a longer period of time. Persistent nasal obstruction on one side only should make one suspect the presence of a foreign object, or perhaps even a tumor.

Asthma that occurs after strenuous exercise is called exercise-induced asthma. Such an attack is usually mild and will disappear after rest.

If a person has been relatively free of asthma until exposure to animals, cut grass, or a virus, and if the exposure is brief, the attack should subside with proper treatment. It may even subside spontaneously.

Itching (Pruritus)   Infants and young children may suffer from a red, flat, scaly rash. Itching is intense and can lead to what is known as "weeping" lesions, caused by the oozing of serum from underlying small blood vessels. Typical places for this to happen are the cheeks, the creases behind the ears, and at the bends of the arms and legs. Commonly called eczema or atopic (allergic) dermatitis, the rash can spread enough to become disabling. During the healing stages, the affected skin thickens and becomes dry and cracked; some bleeding may also occur. A local infection that takes the form of skin boils is serious and should be considered a threat.

Hives   Raised bumps, ranging in size from that of small peas to sizable portions of the body, may appear anywhere on the body. Each lesion may last only a few hours, but new ones can appear at frequent intervals. The itching may become so intense that it is difficult to perform a task or sleep soundly.

Contact Dermatitis   This type of reaction resembles eczema, except that the inflamed skin has sharper borders, does not commonly affect the crease areas, nor does it last as long. Blisters are more likely. Removal and avoidance of the chemical responsible for the blisters will, in most cases, provide relief within two weeks.

Hay Fever   Itching within the nasal passages, a prominent symptom of hay fever, causes nose-rubbing and facial contortions as a person attempts to relieve the misery. The inner corners of the eyes, and even their entire surface, may itch, resulting in tears. Also, itching of the roof of the mouth can be extremely annoying.

Pain   Allergic conjunctivitis can induce a painful, burning condition known as pinkeye. Bright light often adds to the discomfort. Allergic rhinitis, especially in children, may block the Eustachian tubes, which extend from the throat to the middle of the ears. This part of the ear is a closed box devoid of air except for a tiny exit tube that adjusts the ear to pressure changes. When a Eustachian tube is blocked, air is trapped and exerts pressure, resulting in a sharp pain deep within the ears. Known as aerotitis, the condition is sometimes caused by sudden changes of air or water pressure, for example, when one goes up a mountain or dives underwater.

Allergic rhinitis is also associated with serous otitis media, the leakage of fluid into the middle ear. It causes an aching pain that can temporarily diminish hearing. If untreated, the infection can cause fever and increased pain, and lead ultimately to rupture of the eardrum.

In the nasal passages are found outlets from the sinuses—air spaces in the bony structure of the skull. The sinuses near the nose, under the cheeks, and above the eyes (sinuses known, respectively, as ethmoid, maxillary, and frontal) can become obstructed. Buildup of air or fluid leads to greater pressure, which produces pain ranging from a dull ache to a sharp, steady pain around the areas affected. This pain is a symptom of sinusitis.

An asthma attack itself can be painful. Additional movement of the chest wall muscles is felt either as a heavy weight on the chest or as tightness. If the complications of pneumothorax, rib fracture, or pneumonia occur, the pain becomes more pronounced, resembling breathing in pleurisy.

Although none of these illnesses is life-threatening, any one of them can become troublesome enough to interfere with one's normal life. They should not, however, cause undue fear or send one to a hospital emergency room. Prompt attention and appropriate medication are a better response.

Coping with Emergencies and Other Less Serious Allergic Conditions

Proper management of an allergy requires proper diagnosis. Whenever possible, an illness should first be diagnosed and evaluated by a physician, preferably by a family physician or the physician primarily responsible for treatment. The physician may request confirmation or further evaluation from a qualified allergist trained in, for example, pediatrics or internal medicine. The specialist may be a clinical immunologist whose subspecialty is allergy. A patient whose illness involves only one body system may be evaluated by a specialist in, say, diseases of the ear, nose, and throat; the chest; or the skin. In a case requiring laboratory tests, the services of an immunopathologist may be needed.

The physician responsible for directing a person's health care should make a diagnosis, estimate the specific causes, and prescribe a program of treatment. People tend to become allergic to substances that cannot be avoided entirely, short of withdrawing from society. Thus, the more they know about the causes, or precipitating factors, of allergies, and how to avoid them, the less the risk of recurrence. In general, the following apply to all allergy emergencies.

You should know:

The names of all medications known to cause an allergic reaction or have a severe side effect

The allergen or allergens that caused the reaction or side effect

The season or seasons in which pollen caused the symptoms that are most prevalent—for example, early spring (trees), spring and early summer (grasses), or fall (weeds and certain trees)

The names and doses of all medications, professionally prescribed and self-prescribed, including vitamins, "health foods," and cold tablets

Related families of the drugs and allergens that are known reactors

You should keep a written record of

Drug reactions; consider using a Medic Alert bracelet, an identity bracelet, "dog tags," or a drug-information card.

Current drug therapy; everyone on steroid treatment for more than a few weeks should carry a card with a message such as: *I am taking steroids* [specific name and dose] *on a regular basis. Do not stop dosage in case of a serious accident or major surgery.* The name and phone number of your physician should also be listed.

Allergens other than drugs—for instance, stinging insects, dust, mold, pets, food.

The location of emergency-room facilities near your home, place of work, and other places you are likely to be.

Emergencies may be inadvertently self-induced. Use of the following list will help prevent them:

Take steroids as prescribed.

Treat asthma adequately until it is fully resolved.

Inform medical personnel about known reactions to drugs.

Avoid known allergens and irritants.

Do not overdose or overuse medications.

It is senseless, and possibly tragic, to casually reexpose oneself to a drug, x-ray, or preparation known to have caused an anaphylactic reaction in the past. The only exception is when both a person and that person's physician agree that not taking the substance would be more dangerous than taking it. Once the risks have been evaluated, effective preexposure-treatment measures can usually be taken. Tragedies occur when reexposure occurs because of oversight or carelessness.

It is the physician's responsibility to inquire about past reactions to drugs and solutions used in x-ray studies; it is the patient's responsibility to provide such information. Carrying a drug-information card or wearing an information bracelet makes allowance for the possibility of loss of consciousness or other inability to communicate.

Self-medication is especially risky for allergic people. If a certain medication causes a serious reaction, it is likely that another chemically similar drug bearing a different name will behave similarly. For example, penicillin is related to drugs with different names such as cephalosporin and Keflex. Ordinarily, it is not possible to learn all the drug families. You should ask your physician whether a preparation about to be administered is related to the one that caused the allergic reaction. If you insist on self-medication, however, you should know as much as possible about the chemicals used in non-prescription medications and the equivalent terms of these ingredients. If, in the past, aspirin caused hives, asthma, or an anaphylactoid reaction, so will acetylsalicylic acid, for it and aspirin are the same chemically.

A similar situation exists in the case of foods. Merely a taste of peanuts or lobster can cause anaphylaxis in the highly susceptible person. The peanut is a legume; therefore, such legumes as peas and beans must be considered potentially hazardous. If you are allergic to crustaceans, and you know that lobster is a crustacean, you will want to avoid its close relatives, crabs and shrimps. Clams and oysters, popularly thought of as shellfish, too, are actually mollusks, differing both chemically and antigenically.

Let us now consider the medical conditions on an individual basis, from emergency to nonemergency reactions.

Emergency Reactions

Anaphylaxis

Any person who has suffered an anaphylactic reaction—whether to a food, insect sting, drug, or medical procedure—is susceptible to other attacks. Although an anaphylactic reaction may never recur, that person cannot be certain of always avoiding concealed food, a drug accidentally administered, a medical procedure, or the sudden sting of an insect.

Once an anaphylactic reaction begins, the best treatment is an injection of epinephrine (Adrenalin). The drug works within minutes, tightening the blood vessels to prevent serum from escaping, and thus preventing edema. The same action tends to maintain blood pressure while acting simultaneously to keep the airways open. The injection procedure is not difficult to learn. Before prescribing the self-medication of Adrenalin, a physician should demonstrate its proper use and allow the patient to practice the self-injection procedure.

First-aid kits containing epinephrine (the generic name for Adrenalin) are available in various forms. The Emergency Ana-Kit (manufactured by Hollister-Stier in Spokane, Washington) contains 1 preloaded syringe containing a 0.3-milliliter (5 milliliters equals 1 teaspoon) dose of epinephrine in a red plastic box 4½ inches long, one and three-fourths inches wide, and an inch deep; four chewable doses of the antihistamine Chlorpheniramine (2 milligrams each) in a sealed, clear plastic wrap; two wrapped, isopropyl alcohol swabs, and a thin string-type tourniquet. The Insect Sting First Aid Kit, sold by Center Laboratories in Port Washington, New York, is a box approximately 6 by 2¼ by 1 inch and containing a prefilled syringe containing a 1:1,000 solution of epinephrine, an alcohol pad, a tourniquet, antihistamine tablets of Chlorpheniramine (4 milligrams each), and 2 ephedrine-phenobarbital tablets. Some other manufacturers market prefilled syringes of epinephrine, which can be injected automatically (Epi. Pen. Center Laboratories).

The needle is injected into the fatty tissue under the skin—not in a muscle, vein, or artery. The usual dose is 0.3 milliliter of a 1:1,000 solution of epinephrine. It is best to administer a smaller dose, preferably 0.2 milliliter, to patients under age seven, to those who weigh less than forty pounds, or to adults with heart irregularities or coronary vessel disease.

This step is followed by taking an antihistamine tablet. Among adults, 50 milligrams of Benadryl or 4 of Chlortrimeton (Chlorpheniramine) is commonly used. Children under the age of seven should take half this dosage. If an anaphylactic reaction has not begun to subside within twenty minutes, the dose should be repeated.

Epinephrine is also available in a metered, self-administered aerosol activated by hand while the user inhales. Such preparations as Medihalor-Epi, manufactured by Riker Laboratories in Northridge, California, are available without prescription. Although not a substitute for injectable epinephrine in cases of anaphylaxis, Medihalor-Epi may be helpful as a backup treatment for the throat (laryngeal edema) or for bronchial swelling (asthma), either of which may occur alone or as a manifestation of anaphylaxis. Portable and virtually indestructible, these devices can be carried in automobiles, briefcases, handbags, and so on.

The kits should be checked every month to make sure the clear epinephrine solution has not discolored (usually becoming amber). Such change, accelerated by sunlight, indicates decreased potency. The aerosol should be activated periodically to determine whether the valve opening is still free of dust. If it is not, cleaning with soapy water or ammonia will remove the dust.

If an allergen—for example, food or medicine—causing the anaphylaxis has been ingested, remove as much of the material as possible by spitting or rinsing it out, making sure that you do not swallow. If necessary, vomiting can usually be induced by placing one or two fingers at the rear of the mouth.

If the allergen has been injected into the arm, a tourniquet should be applied tightly between the site of the injection and the shoulder. Tourniquets are available in first-aid kits, or they can be purchased separately or improvised from shoestrings, cord, or large rubber bands. Tourniquets placed between the injection site and the heart will slow the absorption and circulation of such allergens as bee or wasp venom.

Insect Stings　An integral part of coping with allergic emergencies is their prevention. Regarding stinging insects, the following information should be helpful. It has been prepared by the American Academy of Allergy and is excerpted with the academy's permission. Obviously, people who are allergic to bees, hornets, wasps, or yellow jackets should do everything practicable to avoid being stung. The chance of being stung can be lessened by taking the simple precautions described in the following paragraphs.

Preventive methods at home　Food attracts the Hymenoptera

(bees, hornets, wasps, and yellow jackets), as do outdoor cooking and eating, feeding pets outdoors, and partially filled garbage cans. Even dribble from a child's popsicle will attract insects. Keeping food covered until the moment of disposal, meticulous cleanliness about garbage areas, and the occasional spraying of patio and garbage cans with insecticides will contribute to keeping insects away. Gardening should be done cautiously. Cutting the grass with a scythe or sling blade, running a power mower over an underground yellow jacket nest, penetrating a bumble bee's nest with a trowel, and clipping a hedge are all risky activities for people sensitive to insect stings. Finally, vines that can conceal nests or hives should be removed.

Personal methods of prevention   Perfume, hairspray, hair tonic, suntan lotion, and many other cosmetics attract insects. Loose clothing in which insects might become trapped, bright colors, flowery prints, and the color black should all be avoided. Light colors—for example, white, green, tan, and khaki—are not considered attractive or antagonistic to bees. Any object, no matter how lightly it is touched, should be checked first for bees, hornets, wasps, or yellow jackets. Children should be taught not to pick up a wagon handle (or any toy, for that matter) without first looking for an insect on it. For instance, idly kicking a rotted log can send vibrations into the ground that disturb nearby yellow jackets. Public trash cans should be avoided. An insecticide bomb kept in a car's glove compartment may be used when a stray insect flies in. Shoes or sneakers should be worn at all times when one is outdoors. Even hard beach sand should be suspect; one type of wasp spends most of its life on dune grass. Sandals do not provide adequate protection.

Immediate removal of a stinger   The honeybee is the only insect that leaves its stinger (with venom sac attached) in the victim. Because it takes two to three minutes for all the venom to be injected, quick removal of the stinger and the sac will prevent much of the poison's harmful effect. This is done with one swift scrape of the fingernail. The sac should not be picked up between thumb and forefinger; that merely squeezes in more venom. Hornets, wasps, and yellow jackets do not lose their stinger and should be brushed off promptly. Although some Hymenoptera are more combative than others, any insect will sting if its hive is disturbed. Thus, while it is important to destroy hives and nests, this should never be done by or in the presence of someone who is allergic to Hymenoptera. Instead, a hive or nest should be removed by an exterminator or at least by someone not allergic to stings.

Nests and their removal   Wasps build open-comb nests under eaves, behind shutters, in carports, shrubs, and woodpiles—in fact, almost any place that is protected. Nests can be destroyed by hosing, carefully knocking them down with a stick or broom handle, or scraping them into a jar (which should then be covered quickly). The area should be sprayed with an insecticide once daily for two to three days to discourage rebuilding at the same site. Jet sprays can reach twelve to fifteen feet. Yellow jackets build in the ground and emerge through a small hole, which should be marked during the day with a thin stick. At dusk, when all the insects have returned for the night, a liberal amount of gasoline, lye, or kerosene should be poured into the hole. Do not light the gasoline or kerosene, though. This procedure should be repeated the next evening to make sure the fumes have thoroughly penetrated the holes. A water hose should never be pointed at the hole; that will merely cause the insects to attack the person holding the hose. Hornets build a gray hive shaped like a football, usually in a shrub or high in a tree. If you can't reach the nest with a flame or trap the insects in a jar, bucket, or metal drum, a pest exterminator or the fire department should be called in.

Whether swarming on a twig or nesting in a hollow tree, honeybees may be removed by following one or more of the methods described above. They can also be removed by a beekeeper, who is frequently glad to acquire another colony. When a nest is out of reach, help from the fire department or a county agent of the Department of Agriculture should be considered.

In conclusion, the allergic person should use common sense—keep calm and act quickly, avoid situations in which insects have been known to attack, and keep a sharp lookout when outdoors.

Laryngeal Edema

The condition known as laryngeal edema is usually part of the multiple involvement of anaphylaxis; occasionally, it may be the sole reaction to a food, drug, or sting. The best remedy is to inject epinephrine, as described above; the next best thing to do is inhale two doses from an epinephrine aerosol, supplemented by oral antihistamine tablets. Normally, the condition improves within minutes; if it does not, suffocation, cyanosis (bluish skin caused by lack of air), and loss of consciousness will occur. If the throat or the lower windpipe remains closed despite self-medication, medical attention should be sought immediately. During the approximately five minutes available before permanent damage results from lack of oxygen, a surgical procedure known as a tracheotomy must be performed. The procedure consists of making an opening in the windpipe below the obstructed area, to allow oxygen to enter the lungs. Another medical procedure, called cardiopulmonary resuscitation, is sometimes used, but the procedure is not effective if air cannot be forced through the obstructed windpipe.

Asthma

The injection of epinephrine is, with only a few exceptions, the treatment of choice. Alternatives should be sought if an epinephrine or epinephrine-type aerosol has been inhaled four or more times within the preceding hour, or if the heartbeat is extremely fast and irregular. (A fast but regular heartbeat, or a moderate increase in high blood pressure, should not deter one from injecting epinephrine if an asthma attack is becoming more severe.)

If prescribed drugs have not been taken up to the dosage level allowed, they should be taken to that level before resorting to injections. Two tablets of Tedral, Marax, or a similar combination drug can be tolerated without serious side effects in an otherwise healthy adult with a severe asthma attack. Similarly, the following drugs may be taken safely: up to two tablets of metaproterenol (Alupent and Metaprel), 10 milligrams each; terbutaline (Bricanyl and Brethine), 5 milligrams each; or one of the standard (not long-acting) theophylline preparations, up to 250 milligrams. Depending on someone's prior experience, he or she may be able to tolerate single doses of both the adrenergic and the theophylline drugs taken together. If nausea or vomiting precludes oral therapy, an inhaled or injected bronchodilator is the next treatment. An acute asthma attack is not the time for treatment with inhaled cromolyn (Intal) or beclomethasone (Vanceril and Beclovent); these are designed for prevention. A person regularly taking prescribed steroid drugs such as prednisone, who has omitted one or more doses, should take the amount missed immediately. Many physicians prescribe extra doses of steroids in treating attacks of asthma that are increasing in severity. Consult your physician ahead of time about what you should do in case of worsening asthma or for a sudden, severe attack in cases where medical attention is not readily available.

It is most important that you become familiar with all asthma medication. Know the name, amount (usually given in milligrams, abbreviated "mg" if in tablet or capsule form, and "mg per ml" if liquid), and frequency of dosage. It is equally important that you regularly monitor medication to ensure an adequate supply, and that the expiration date printed on the label has not passed. Keep medications only in clearly labeled containers—with names, directions for use, and expiration dates. Because one occasionally forgets, the location and business hours of the nearest pharmacy should be kept handy.

Prevention is still the most effective treatment for asthma. Try to anticipate when and where asthma will be aggravated, so you can take measures to avoid these times and places and increase medication. Because asthma can get out of control fairly rapidly, you should not ignore attacks that are worsening; neither should you test the limit of your tolerance. You should, of course, avoid anything that can aggravate asthma. The careful asthma victim will fully and quickly treat an attack with prescribed medication, thus avoiding in most cases, discomfort, emergency room treatment, and hospitalization.

Skin Reactions

Eczema and contact dermatitis are lesions that have become inflamed. In the early stages of inflammation, the lesions should be cleaned carefully with cool water, baking soda or cornstarch soaks, or with a nonperfumed lotion. Avoid excessive exposure to water, heavy ointments, and heat, since these tend to smother the skin and cause it to dry out, thus adding to the inflammation. A solution or lotion containing steroids for the skin usually speeds the healing process. These preparations are usually prescription items. Avoid using antibiotic or antihistamine creams, which can increase the sensitivity. If itching is a problem—as it often is—the best relief is through the use of oral antihistamines.

In the late stages of eczema, the skin becomes tender, swollen, and less red while some scaling of tissue occurs. The itchy scales can be removed with a cotton swab moistened with olive or mineral oil. Lotions may be changed to creams, particularly those containing steroids. If the itching continues, antihistamines should be taken every six to eight hours. In cases that do not respond to this treatment, healing is usually aided by steroids taken orally or by injection. Such therapy, however, must be supervised by a physician.

Prevention is important in this group of skin diseases. The allergens involved can often be identified, and should be carefully avoided. The most common allergens that cause eczema are foods such as milk and other dairy products (infants are particularly sensitive), eggs, oranges, and wheat products. Contact dermatitis is caused by the resins of such plants as poison ivy, poison oak, sumac, primrose, and ragweed, as well as by chemicals in cosmetics, clothing, shoes, and jewelry. Hives can be provoked by drugs, especially penicillin, aspirin, codeine, and certain foods. Other causes of hives are parasitic worm infections and insect stings. Some people develop hives from physical pressure on the skin or from extremes of hot or cold. Although the causes of many forms of eczema and hives are not yet known, you should make a concerted effort to identify the causes, and thus prevent a recurrence.

People suffering from colds, skin infections, chicken pox, or herpes viral infections should be avoided, since their organisms can contaminate allergic dermatitis.

Because hives are often generalized, and the skin covering them is intact, the use of skin preparations will have less effect than when they are used for eczema or contact dermatitis. Itching and swelling usually respond well to oral antihistamines. Ephedrine, an adrenergic drug available in 25-milligram doses without prescription, is used to reduce the swelling. If hives increase, and if angioedema is severe, injectable epinephrine should be taken. A dose of 0.2 to 0.3 milliliter of epinephrine 1:1,000 injected subcutaneously, as in asthma or anaphylaxis, is recommended.

Nonemergency Reactions

Nasal Stuffiness

Following are some suggestions for the relief of less serious allergic reactions:

1. Oral nasal decongestant drugs such as pseudoephedrine may be taken up to four times daily in doses of 30 to 60 milligrams each.

2. Nasal passages may be irrigated with a mild salt solution made with four ounces of warm tap water and a quarter teaspoon of table salt, using a nasal dropper.

3. Nose drops and sprays—for example, Neosynephrine, phenylephrine, Afrin, or other long-acting medication—should not be used for more than four consecutive days. Chronic use leads to renewed swelling and nasal obstruction, caused by the drops. Nasal solutions containing Mentholatum and other oils are best avoided.

4. For temporary relief, take hot showers and apply heating pads and hot cloths to the nasal area.

Sneezing, Itching, and Watery Discharge of Hay Fever

Antihistamines are more effective in relieving the itch and watery discharge phases of hay fever and allergic rhinitis. If a person is taking blood-pressure medications such as reserpine or propanalol, a physician should be consulted as to whether the medications are contributing to the stuffiness. The following suggestions should help relieve symptoms:

1. An antihistamine is the best choice of drug. Chlorphenera-mine, in doses of 2 and 4 milligrams, are obtainable without a prescription. Such side effects as drowsiness, dryness, and gastric disturbance can be combated by varying either the dose or the preparation. Many preparations are combinations of antihistamines and adrenergic decongestants. For rapid, reliable action, a short-acting drug is preferable. Among many people, "sustained-effect" drugs are absorbed less evenly; they may be considered for night-time use after other symptoms have been controlled.

2. Avoidance measures should be considered part of the treatment. If the culprit is pollen, exposure should be minimized. Avoid gardening, lawn mowing, and hiking in areas of tall vegetation. Stay indoors during high winds and keep bedroom windows closed when sleeping. If conditions at work produce symptoms, consider such measures as improving the ventilation, installing suction air hoods, and using a respiratory mask.

Pain from Sinusitis and Middle-Ear Allergy

The following may be used to relieve the pain of sinusitis or middle-ear allergy:

1. Nasal decongestants, whether used locally or orally, help open clogged tubes to the sinus cavities and the middle-ear chambers.

2. Heat applied to the local sinus area and the ears—in the form of a heating pad, hot cloths, or warm mineral oil solution in the ears—provides some relief.

3. Medications for pain—such as aspirin and acetaminophen (Tylenol and Valadol)—may be taken until medical attention can be obtained.

4. Antihistamines can be used to treat the underlying allergic rhinitis.

5. Avoid swimming, diving, and trips to high elevations until the condition improves.

Summary

Allergy emergencies are not common, and they are rarely fatal. Those that do require immediate attention are anaphylaxis, a generalized, allergic shocklike reaction; laryngeal, or tracheal, edema (swelling of the windpipe); and severe asthma, or bronchospasm. Epinephrine by injection is the drug of choice in all three emergencies. Although allergy emergencies have numerous causes, a general knowledge of them can enable the allergy sufferer to prevent recurrences. Other related allergic illnesses, while discomforting and sometimes alarming, are not life-threatening. Self-treatment measures are available to provide relief until more extensive medical attention can be obtained.

Allergy emergencies can be treated successfully, and some can often be prevented. Unlike some injuries and certain illnesses, the outlook for complete recovery is good.

CHAPTER 4

Allergic Diseases
and Their Treatment
by Thomas M. Golbert, M.D.

The drugs used in treating allergic disorders are categorized broadly as antihistamines, decongestants, bronchodilators, bischromones, expectorants, or corticosteroids. Another category—immunosuppressives—which inhibit the immune system, have been tested but are not yet recommended for use. This chapter will review some of the medications commonly used to relieve allergic disorders.

Antihistamines

Uses

Antihistamines are used in treating various disorders of the stomach and intestines (the gastrointestinal tract) and of the nose and skin. They are particularly effective in the treatment of hay fever (allergic rhinitis) and other inflammations of the nose (vasomotor rhinitis and intrinsic rhinitis); of hives (urticaria); contact dermatitis; eczema; allergic rashes similar to measles; and allergic reactions in the stomach and intestines (gastrointestinal allergy). The itching associated with rashes such as eczema and contact dermatitis is decreased, although the appearance of the rash often is not immediately altered. Antihistamines are also used to supplement the treatment of allergic reactions or reactions similar to those of allergies which involve more than one body system (for example, the lungs and the skin). These reactions are known medically as systemic allergic reactions or idiosyncratic reactions (reactions similar to systemic allergic reactions, but in which allergic mechanisms cannot be demonstrated).

In general, antihistamines are not effective in treating asthma, although some asthma patients may benefit from treatment with these drugs.

Representative Drugs

The antihistamines used to treat allergic disorders are commonly divided into six classes, with the following chemical names: ethanolamine, ethylenediamine, alkylamine, piperazine, and phenothiazine. The sixth class is a group of miscellaneous compounds. Drugs classified as members of the first five classes are chemically related; those in class VI are not necessarily related chemically to each other, nor to members of the five other classes. The drugs in classes I through V have therapeutic properties similar to those of other drugs in the same class. Although patients vary in their responses to specific drugs, their reactions to various chemically related preparations are similar. Sometimes a patient develops a tolerance to an antihistamine drug, which renders the antihistamine ineffective for that patient. This phenomenon is usually dealt with by switching to a chemically unrelated antihistamine, or by discontinuing an antihistamine for awhile, which removes the tolerance for that antihistamine.

Class I antihistamines—the ethanolamines—are the most potent antihistamines in terms of therapeutic equivalents. This group includes: bromodiphenhydramine; dimenhydrinate (Dramamine and Ambodryl); carbinoxamine (Clistin and Clistin R.A.); clemastine (Tavist); diphenhydramine (Baramine, Benadryl, and SK-Diphenhydyramine); diphenylpyraline (Diafen and Hispril); and doxylamine (Decapryn).

Class II, the ethylenediamines, includes: methapyrilene (Histadyl); pyrilamine (Histalon, Neo-Antergan, Neo-Pyramine, and Nisaval); and tripelennamine (Pyribenzamine, Pbz, and Pbz-SR).

Class III, the alkylamines, contains probably the most commonly prescribed antihistamines. Representative compounds are: brompheniramine (Dimetane and Dimetane Extentabs); chlorpheniramine (sold under numerous trade names); dexbrompheniramine (Disomer Chronotabs); dexchlorpheniramine (Polaramine and Polaramine Repetabs); dimethindine (Forhistal, Forhistal Lontabs, Triten, and Triten Tab-In); and triprolidine (Actidil).

Some ethylenediamines and alkylamines are available without prescription. They are also available in many nonprescription, fixed-dose combinations marketed as compounds for the relief of colds, hay fever, and headaches.

Class IV consists of piperazines and includes cyclizine (Marezine) and meclizine (Bonine). Drugs in this group, along with dimenhydrinate in class I, are used primarily for treating motion sickness.

Phenothiazines make up class V. Representative drugs are methdilazine (Tacaryl), promethazine (Phenergan), and trimeprazine (Temaril). Phenothiazines are used principally as tranquilizers, although they also have antihistaminic properties, which make them useful in relieving rashes.

Class VI, a group of miscellaneous compounds, includes the chemically related azatadine (Optimine) and cyproheptadine (Periactin). Both compounds inhibit the neurotransmitter serotonin, as well as histamine, and are used mostly to alleviate the itching common in skin disorders. Cyproheptadine may be helpful in treating hives caused by exposure to low temperatures (cold urticaria). The hydroxyzines (Atarax and Vistaril) are related most closely to the piperazines. Hydroxyzine, used primarily for treating allergic rashes, has recently been demonstrated as beneficial in the relief of hay fever in some patients; it is also useful as a tranquilizer.

Many fixed-ratio combinations of two or more antihistamines, or of antihistamines plus decongestants, are widely used.

Another group of antihistamines, the H2 antihistamines, have vastly different treatment properties. Cimetidine (known by the trade name Tagamet) is, however, the only member of this group approved by the Food and Drug Administration, having been approved for treating peptic ulcers but not allergic disorders. Some studies indicate that a combination of cimetidine and an antihistamine from one of the other groups may be more effective than other antihistamines alone in treating some cases of hives that last more than three months (chronic urticaria). Theoretically, cimetidine should not be used alone in the treatment of allergic disorders.

Side Effects and Precautions

Side effects are rarely serious among the drugs in groups I through VI when they are used in therapeutic doses; side effects that do occur disappear with prolonged use. Sometimes, though, a drug must be discontinued or the dosage reduced. Reactions to these drugs vary markedly, but most patients do not experience bothersome side effects. The most common side effect is drowsiness, especially when phenothiazines and ethanolamines are used. Ethylenediamines usually have a moderately sedative effect, whereas alkylamines generally have the least sedative effect.

Abdominal symptoms are the next most common side effect. They include upper abdominal discomfort, nausea, vomiting, loss of appetite, and constipation or diarrhea. Relief from some of these effects may be obtained by taking the drug with meals. These effects occur most often when ethylenediamines are used, and least often when ethanolamines or alkylamines are used.

Other side effects are a dry mouth and throat, frequent and/or painful urination, awareness of rapid heartbeat, headache, low blood pressure (hypotension), and tightness of the chest. Restlessness, nervousness, inability to sleep, and other manifestations of stimulation of the central nervous system occur occasionally, most often when alkylamines are used. Symptoms of anxiety—such as heavy, tingling, or weak hands—may also appear. Stimulation of the central nervous system is a striking feature in antihistamine poisoning, symptoms of which may be excitement, hallucinations, lack of coordination, and convulsions. Rare side effects are difficulty urinating, impotence, allergic rashes, and aggravation of already existing high blood pressure. Reduction of the blood cell count, an extremely rare complication, is reversible.

Other side effects of phenothiazines are jaundice resulting from obstructions in the biliary tract, blood abnormalities, sunlight-sensitivity rashes, tremors, and impairment of the central nervous system's control of posture and movement.

Antihistamines can enhance the effects of alcohol and of tranquilizers, barbiturates, and other sedatives. They should not be used with "mood elevators" (antidepressant drugs) of the monoamine oxidase (MAO) inhibitor type. Some antihistamines counter the effects of such drugs as guanethidine, used to treat high blood pressure.

Piperazines should not be used during pregnancy. Cyproheptadine should not be given to premature or newborn infants. It has also been reported to cause weight gain.

The most common adverse effects of cimetidine are diarrhea, dizziness, muscle pain, and rash. Confusion and symptoms of central nervous system disorders have occurred in elderly patients whose kidneys were not functioning properly. These effects, usually associated with excessive doses, disappeared after the patients stopped taking the drug.

In some tests, abnormal liver function (serum transaminase and, rarely, alkaline phosphatase) has been reported. A small increase in the serum creatinine level may occur without other evidence of kidney dysfunction, and a rare form of drug-induced kidney disease known as interstitial nephritis has been observed. These abnormalities, however, have been removed by discontinuing the drug.

Enlarged breasts (gynecomastia) in men, as well as swollen and tender nipples, have been noted, but with no evidence of endocrine dysfunction. Some men who have used the drug more than two months have experienced a decreased sperm count. No causal relationship has been established among other adverse effects reported, including a reduced peripheral white blood cell count, inhibition of delayed immune responses after six weeks of treatment, fever, and slow heart rate (bradycardia).

Since the main route of excretion of cimetidine is through the kidneys, the dose must be reduced in patients suffering from impaired kidney function. Cimetidine increases the activity of "blood thinners," warfarinlike anticoagulants commonly prescribed to inhibit blood clotting. Because the drug crosses the placenta, its safety during pregnancy is questionable.

Decongestants

Uses

Decongestants are used primarily in the treatment of hay fever, vasomotor rhinitis, and intrinsic rhinitis. They also provide some relief of allergy of the stomach and intestines (gastrointestinal allergy) and occasionally of hives. For treating hives, however, drugs such as epinephrine and ephedrine are used more widely.

Representative Drugs

Pseudoephedrine hydrochloride (D-Feda, Novafed, and Sudafed) are probably the most widely used oral decongestants. Others are ephedrine, phenylephrine, phenylpropanolamine (Propadrine), and pseudoephedrine sulfate (Afrinol). Ephedrine, which stimulates the central nervous system more than do such drugs as pseudoephedrine, is used primarily as a bronchodilator. Pseudoephedrine has fewer side effects than ephedrine. Although it is active as a bronchodilator, it is less effective than other drugs in treating asthma. Commonly used intranasal preparations are naphazoline (Privine), oxymetazoline (Afrin), phenylephrine (Neo-Synephrine), tetrahydrozoline (Tyzine), and zymetazoline (Otrivin).

Side Effects and Precautions

Among the side effects of oral preparations, as well as the effects of overdoses of intranasal preparations, are nervousness, dizziness, nausea, awareness of heartbeat (usually rapid), and occasionally stimulation of the central nervous system. Other effects, which usually occur among children, are high blood pressure, slow heart rate, irregular heart rhythm, and low blood pressure. Children have also been known to experience severe side effects, including sweating, drowsiness, deep sleep, coma, hypotension, and slow heart rate. Because of the effects listed above, caution should be exercised when these drugs are used in people with heart disease, high blood pressure, sugar diabetes, thyroid disease, or any combination of these diseases, or those taking drugs (also known as "mood elevators") of the tricyclic class. Patients taking the monoamine oxidase (MAO) inhibitor class of antidepressive drugs should not also use decongestant drugs.

Intranasal agents require additional precautions. For example, they should be used only in treating illnesses that are short and relatively severe, that is, illnesses that do not exceed five days in duration. Prolonged use often causes a "rebound" phenomenon in which, while more and more of the drug is required, the desired effect of the drug becomes increasingly less. More frequent and larger doses of a drug are used, accompanied by the twin risks of overdose and toxicity. Prolonged use causes rhinitis medicamentosum, a condition in which the mucous membranes of the nasal passages become red, boggy, or pale gray and edematous (swelling with fluid between the cells) and in which the inflamed membranes are indistinguishable from other forms of chronic inflammation of the nose, such as year-round hay fever (perennial allergic rhinitis). Topical nasal decongestant solutions quickly become contaminated with bacteria and fungi after use, and for this reason, may be sources of infection. Some rules to follow in using spray decongestants are:

1. Rinse the spray tip or dropper in hot water after each use.
2. Do not place the spray tip or dropper inside the nose.
3. Confine use of a particular applicator to one person.
4. Discard the medication and its container when the medication is no longer needed.

Something over which people have no control, but which they should be aware of, is that most topical nasal decongestant solutions interact with aluminum and thus should not be stored in containers made wholly or in part of the metal.

Bronchodilators

Uses

Bronchodilators are used primarily in treating asthma, but they are also used to treat chronic bronchitis and emphysema, diseases of the lung which chronically obstruct the air passages, as well as to treat bronchiectasis, in which dilatations occur in the air passages of the lungs. Some bronchodilators are useful in alleviating several forms of hives. Epinephrine was the first drug chosen for treating allergic or allergylike responses involving more than one body system, for example, the simultaneous occurrence of hives and asthma. Another bronchodilator is aminophylline, which is useful as a supplemental treatment in some cases of systemic reaction.

Representative Drugs

Three classes of bronchodilators are currently being used: adrenergic agonists (also known as sympathomimetic drugs); methylxanthines; and anticholinergics (also known as parasympatholytic drugs). Anticholinergic drugs are now being tested and have not yet been approved by the Food and Drug Administration. Other drugs now being tested are alpha adrenergic agonists and prostaglandins.

Adrenergic Agonists   All of the following drugs dilate the air passages (the bronchi and bronchioles) of the lungs as well as affecting, in numerous ways, the blood vessels, heart, small intestines, central nervous system, and, in women, the uterus: epinephrine aqueous suspension (Asmolin and Sus-Phrine); epinephrine hydrochloride (Adrenalin Chloride in a 1:1,000 solution for subcutaneous or intramuscular injection; available in 1:100 solution for oral inhalation under many trade names); ephedrine (Ephedrine USP); and ethylnorepinephrine (Bronkephrine). Epinephrine hydrochloride is often the first drug used in treating allergic or allergylike reactions involving multiple organs. Ephedrine is available for both injection and oral use, but most often it is used orally in one of many fixed-ratio combinations of drugs. Methoxyphenamine, which is similar to ephedrine, is taken orally.

Isoproterenol (available under many trade names) and protokylol (Ventaire) both dilate the air passages of the lungs and affect the blood vessels, heart, small intestines, and, in women, the uterus. Isoproterenol is available for oral inhalation, as a lozenge to be placed under the tongue, and as a 1:5,000 solution for subcutaneous injection. Protokylol is taken orally.

Metaproterenol (Alupent and Metaprel), terbutaline (Brethine and Bricanyl), and salbutamol (Albuterol and Proventil) are relatively selective in dilating the airways of the lung and affecting the blood vessels and the uterus. Metaproterenol has been licensed for use orally or by inhalation. Terbutaline is now available as both an oral and an injectable preparation, and it may soon appear in inhalation form. Salbutamol is available in Europe and some other areas in metered-dose nebulizers for inhalation, but it has not been licensed in the United States.

Methylxanthines The methylxanthines class includes dyphylline (known under various trade names); oxtriphylline (Choledyl); theophylline (known under numerous trade names); and theophylline ethylenediamine or Aminophyllin and aminophylline. Except for dyphylline, all are converted in the body to theophylline.

Anticholinergic The anticholinergic drugs that have been used experimentally are atropine sulfate and ipratropium bromide (SCH-1000). Both are taken by inhalation.

Side Effects and Precautions

Adrenergic Agonists Common side effects of the adrenergic drugs are fear, anxiety, tenseness, restlessness, headache, weakness, tremor, dizziness, pallor, and awareness of heartbeat. They are usually temporary and subside with rest and reassurance. Respiratory difficulty rarely occurs in neurotic patients. Existing symptoms can be aggravated. The most common negative effect of metaproterenol, salbutamol, or terbutaline is tremor. Aggravation of high blood pressure is more likely with drugs that affect the blood vessels and heart, but blood pressure may increase with use of any drug in this group. Metaproterenol, salbutamol, or terbutaline rarely cause low blood pressure. They can also induce nausea, vomiting, and difficulty urinating.

Patients suffering from high blood pressure, thyroid disease, or heart disease should exercise care in using these drugs. Some drugs—those known as cyclopropane or halogenated hydrocarbon anesthetics, which are used to anesthetize patients before surgery—increase the effect of adrenergic agonists on both blood pressure and the heart. Internal cranial bleeding (bleeding inside the head) or abnormal heart rhythm may also occur. Adrenergic agonists are also capable of aggravating diabetes in some patients.

Methylxanthines Irritation of the stomach or intestines, the most common side effects of methylxanthines, can lead to nausea and sometimes to abdominal cramping. Headache and vomiting are associated with excessive doses. Because these drugs stimulate secretion of stomach acid, patients with ulcers of the stomach or intestines should be cautious about using them. Methylxanthines can also affect muscles, which prevent the contents of the stomach from returning to the esophagus through a valvelike mechanism known as the gastroesophageal sphincter, or the cardiac sphincter. Relaxation of this sphincter permits material to flow backward from the stomach into the esophagus.

The use of aminophylline in the form of rectal suppositories results in unpredictable aminophylline blood levels; consequently, their effect in treatment becomes unpredictable. The prolonged use of suppositories can even cause rectal irritation and bleeding. If symptoms of central nervous system stimulation—such as irritability, restlessness, or insomnia—occur, the dose should be reduced. Muscle tremor, or shakiness, may also occur. Overdosage can cause nervous agitation, heightened reflexes, fever, vomiting of blood, convulsions, abnormal heart rhythm, and even death.

Bischromones

Uses

The bischromones, used primarily in treating allergic asthma and exercise-induced asthma, are sometimes used in treating patients with intrinsic asthma. Although bischromones can prevent symptoms of asthma, they should not be used to treat acute, or actively symptomatic, asthma, both because they do not dilate the air passages of the lungs, and because some bischromones are irritants.

Bischromones have been tested for treatment of gastrointestinal allergy as well as some forms of inflammation of the lungs (pneumonia) associated with allergic mechanisms. Dosages of the bischromone cromolyn, used in experimental work, have been as large as 400 milligrams (20 capsules) when taken orally four times a day. Avoiding the food that causes the allergy, however, is safer, simpler, more certain, and much less expensive. Use of the bischromones in studies of various allergic lung diseases has provided researchers with valuable information about the body's immune mechanisms.

Representative Drugs

Cromolyn sodium (Intal) is the only bischromone drug now licensed by the Food and Drug Administration. It is available as a powder in capsule form. Using a special device called a Spin-Haler, the capsule is punctured and the powder is inhaled into the lungs.

Xanthone, another bischromone, is an experimental preparation for oral administration and is not licensed in the United States.

Side Effects and Precautions

Side effects of bischromones occur infrequently. Throat irritation, hoarseness, coughing, and wheezing are the most common. Nausea, vomiting, and dizziness also occur occasionally. Coughing and wheezing often can be prevented by the administration of an aerosolized adrenergic bronchodilator before using cromolyn. Serious but rare side effects are: swelling similar to that of hives under the skin (angioedema); hives; other rashes, allergic reactions involving more than one organ; allergic pneumonia (inflammation of the lungs); gastroenteritis (inflammation of the stomach and intestines); polymyositis (inflamed muscles); and pericarditis (inflammation of the heart covering). These effects subside, however, when use of the drug is discontinued.

The safety of cromolyn when used during pregnancy has not been determined. Studies in animals indicate decreased fetal weight when an animal is given a dose that produces a toxic effect in the mother; but no tumor-producing effect has been reported, even when enormous doses were given intravenously during pregnancy. Potential damaging effects on human fetuses are not known.

Expectorants

Uses

Expectorants promote the removal of mucus from the respiratory tract. They are used in treating asthma and chronic obstructive lung diseases such as chronic bronchitis, emphysema, and bronchiectasis. The last disease named is a condition in which dilatations similar to sacs chronically form in the lungs' air passages.

Representative Drugs

The most widely used expectorants are guaifenesin (glyceril guaiacolate, Robitussin, 2/G, and Glycotuss) and iodides (Potassium Iodide USP and Organidin). Water is still the most effective expectorant, however. Evidence of the effectiveness of other agents is insufficient to justify their use as expectorants; these agents are: ammonium chloride, ipecac, guaiacolsulfonate potassium, and terpin hydrate.

Side Effects and Precautions

No serious side effects from guaifenesin have been reported.

The iodides Potassium Iodide USP and Organidin can cause various allergic manifestations and such side effects as nausea, abdominal cramps, and diarrhea. A group of symptoms called iodism often accompany chronic use; this group usually includes an unpleasant brassy taste, a burning sensation in the mouth and throat, sore teeth and gums, and increased salivation. Other symptoms are: sneezing; runny stuffy nose; eye irritation and swelling of the eyelids; headaches; coughing; a variety of rashes which resemble acne; enlarged painful salivary glands similar to those in mumps; fluid in the lungs (pulmonary edema) and rashes, which may be severe and can on rare occasions cause death. Fever, loss of appetite, and depression, occur occasionally. Iodism usually subsides within a few days after the drug is discontinued. Hypothyroidism, impaired functioning of the thryoid gland, has also been known to occur. Iodides should not be used during pregnancy.

Water intoxication sometimes occurs among people suffering from neurotic or psychotic forms of compulsive drinking, or from certain other diseases. Persons with active asthma or chronic obstructive respiratory diseases, however, usually do not drink enough water.

Corticosteroids

Systemic

Uses Adrenal corticosteroids are effective drugs in treating nearly all allergic disorders. When used over long periods, however, their potential for causing serious side effects limits their usefulness in treating hay fever, eczema, or long-term hives. They are used to relieve acute, chronic asthma that cannot be controlled by other treatment and to treat allergic pneumonia and serum sickness (various combinations of arthritis, rashes, fever, and swollen lymph nodes, or "glands"). Corticosteroids are also used to treat asthma patients who have had to take steroids recently and who now must undergo surgery, or who are having other physical stress. Corticosteroids are sometimes used in cases of acute hives, acute reactions involving multiple organ systems, or for reactions to drugs, serum, or transfusions.

Representative Drugs Corticotropin (ACTH, Acthar, and H.P. Acthar Gel) is a hormone secreted by the pituitary that stimulates the release of cortisone by the adrenal glands. The results of treatment with this drug are unpredictable, though, and it has no advantages over therapy with adrenal corticosteroids or similar drugs.

Cortisone (Cortone) and hydrocortisone (available under several trade names) are fast-acting steroids used briefly during treatment of life-threatening forms of asthma, for reactions involving more than one organ system, and for other acute conditions.

Methylprednisolone (Medrol and Solu-Medrol), prednisolone (available under various trade names), and prednisone (also available under various trade names) are fast-acting preparations that are active over brief periods. Useful in treating acute allergic conditions, they are also suitable for administration on alternate days in cases requiring prolonged therapy. Alternate-day administration has been shown to reduce many adverse effects of prolonged steroid therapy. Depo-Medrol, a long-acting, injectable form of methylprednisolone, is also available.

Cloprednol, another corticosteroid, is active over a shorter period than either methylprednisolone, prednisolone, or prednisone. Yet it may offer the same advantages in alternate-day therapy as the other three. Cloprednol, however, is still experimental and is not licensed by the Food and Drug Administration.

Some long-acting corticosteroid derivatives are betamethasone (Celestone), dexamethasone (available under various trade names), fluprednisolone (Alphadrol), paramethasone acetate (Haldrone), and triamcinolone (Aristocort and Kenacort). These compounds are not suitable for alternate-day therapy.

Side Effects and Precautions The most frequent side effects of corticosteroids are those of water retention and weight gain. In the vast majority of patients, however, these effects aren't severe enough to necessitate stopping the therapy. Other effects are increased susceptibility to bruising, stretch marks, more body hair, insomnia, an inappropriate sense of well-being, leg cramps, an increased number of white blood cells (a condition known as leukocytosis), and a peculiar obesity characterized by a rounded face and thin arms and legs.

More serious complications attributed to corticosteroid therapy are:

Reduced activity of the adrenal glands
Diabetes
High blood pressure
Heart failure

Clots within blood vessels
Inflammation of the arteries (arteritis)
Inflammation of the stomach (gastritis)
Inflammation of the esophagus (esophagitis)
Inflammation of the pancreas (pancreatitis)
Depression of the tissues that produce some of
the white blood cells
Muscle weakness and pain
Rupture of tendons
Thinning of bones
Destruction of bone tissue
Stunted growth in children
Cataracts (which can lead to blindness)
Glaucoma (another cause of blindness)
Protrusion of the eyes
An increase in fungal and viral infections (especially
Herpes species of virus) of the cornea of the eye
Psychosis
Increased pressure within the head
Seizures
Weakness
Increased susceptibility to infection
Increase in body-fat tissue

Peptic ulcer and activation of latent tuberculosis infections have been attributed to corticosteroids, but this is contradicted by recent data. The role of steroids in causing these problems remains controversial.

Corticosteroids usually cause adverse effects only after substantial doses have been administered over extensive periods of time, and most are reversible when the drug is discontinued or the dosage is reduced. There are, however, some irreversible effects, including cataracts and thinning or destruction of bone tissue.

Test results from animal studies *suggest* an increased incidence of fetal malformation, fetal death, and premature birth when corticosteroids are administered to pregnant women, but the data have not been confirmed in humans. The risk of damage to the fetus from lack of oxygen resulting from uncontrolled asthma in the mother seems far greater than from corticosteroid therapy.

Aerosol

Uses Aerosol steroids are topical preparations that are inhaled in the treatment of chronic asthma or sprayed intranasally in treating intractable rhinitis. Whenever it is feasible, topically administered corticosteroids are used to minimize the adverse effects of these drugs.

Representative Drugs   One aerosol steroid used in treating asthma is beclomethasone dipropionate (Beclovent [Becotide in Great Britain and France] and Vanceril). It has also been used experimentally in treating hay fever but is not licensed for this purpose by the Food and Drug Administration. Dexamethasone sodium phosphate (Decadron Turbinaire and Decadron Respihaler) is available for the treatment of hay fever, nasal polyps, and asthma; betamethasone valerate and triamcinolone acetonide are experimental preparations not available in the United States.

Side Effects and Precautions   The most common side effects of aerosol steroid preparations are dry mouth and hoarseness, which usually disappear promptly when the drug is discontinued. The major side effects are fungal infections (called Candida albicans or Aspergillus niger) of the mouth, the pharynx (upper air passages), or occasionally the larynx (voice box). These effects often can be prevented by rinsing the mouth with water each time the medication is taken. Discontinuing the aerosol or treating the infection with an antifungal drug nearly always relieves the condition. On rare occasions, rashes occur, and cataracts have been reported but are considered rare.

Replacing prednisone or other orally administered corticosteroids with aerosol corticosteroids whenever possible is an effective way to reduce the side effects of the former. The adrenal glands, however, stop producing natural hormones during treatment with oral corticosteroids. This effect, called adrenal suppression, does not subside for months after all external sources of corticosteroids (those administered orally, by injection, or, to a lesser extent, by inhalation into the lungs, spraying into the nose, or application to the skin) have been removed. Although the adrenal hormones (to which corticosteroids are related chemically) are harmful in large doses over long periods, they are necessary in small amounts for many body functions. For some functions, the body may be without an adequate supply of adrenal hormones between the time oral corticosteroids are discontinued and the time the adrenal glands resume normal production. This inadequacy—called adrenal insufficiency—is a major concern when aerosol corticosteroids replace oral corticosteroids.

Topical Skin

Uses   Creams, gels, and ointments containing corticosteroids are useful in treating various rashes, particularly eczema and contact dermatitis.

Representative Preparations The most potent preparations (available in a variety of corresponding trade names) are desoximetasone, fluocinolone acetonide acetate, and halcinonide; others are betamethasone, desonide, dexamethasone, flumethasone, fluocinolone acetonide, fluoromethalone, flurandrenolide, hydrocortisone, methylprednisolone, prednisolone, and triamcinolone.

Side Effects and Precautions Complications in the use of topical steroids occur in proportion to their potency, concentration, or frequency and duration of use. When complications do occur, they usually take the form of burning sensations, irritation, itching, dryness, inflammation of the hair follicles, acne, loss of pigmentation, thinning of the skin, stretch marks, a tendency to bruise easily, dilated blood vessels in the skin, and skin ulcers. The risk of infection increases when the area treated is covered with a heavy dressing or a plastic wrap. Topical steroids should be avoided in cases of chicken pox and cowpox (vaccinia). The usual symptoms of scabies infestation (an easily transmitted skin disease, commonly known as mange and characterized by itching), as well as some fungal infections, may be obscured. Contact dermatitis can result when certain preservatives are used.

Ophthalmic

Uses Ophthalmic corticosteroids are useful in treating allergic conjunctivitis (an inflammation of the eye covering) and certain forms of nonallergic, noninfectious conjunctivitis that do not respond to oral antihistamines or topical decongestants.

Representative Preparations Various products are available, including dexamethasone (Decadron), fluorometholone (FML), hydrocortisone (Optef), medrysone (HMS), prednisolone acetate (Prednefrin), and prednisolone sodium phosphate (Inflamase).

Side Effects and Precautions As is true of other corticosteroids, adverse effects depend on the potency, concentration, and frequency and duration of use. Ophthalmic steroid preparations should be avoided in eye infections. Common adverse effects are discomfort and a burning sensation, sometimes accompanied by watery eyes, dilated pupils, blurring of near vision, and drooped eyelids. The bloodstream absorbs enough corticosteroid to cause partial adrenal suppression in adults and, with prolonged use in children, the development of systemic side effects.

Prolonged use of corticosteroids may increase pressure within the eyes and eventually damage the optic nerve, as well as lead to cataracts and, rarely, inflammation of various parts of the eyes.

Summary

The drugs used in treating allergic disorders are considered among the safest in medicine, even though these drugs can have minor side effects, for example, nausea, drowsiness, and nervousness. The more serious side effects occur only rarely, and are usually reversible by discontinuing the drug being used or by reducing the dosage. No drug produces only the precise effect desired; all drugs have various effects. Undesirable effects—called side effects, adverse effects, or secondary effects—become acceptable if the potential therapeutic benefit is sufficient. The potential benefits may be maximized and the risks minimized if drugs are taken as directed by one's physician.

CHAPTER 5

Immunology–The Basic Science of Allergy
by David A. Levy, M.D.

The body's immunologic mechanisms are central to what are commonly regarded as allergic diseases. In order to properly diagnose and manage these diseases and the immunologic reactions to them, we must first have some idea of what immunology is. Immunology deals with the organs, cells, and molecules responsible for recognizing and disposing of foreign (or "nonself") substances that enter the body, with the response to these substances, with interactions between the products of the response and the substances, and with the means of manipulating a response to therapeutic advantage.

The science of immunology arose from a need to study the body's resistance to infection. This resistance is made possible by two types of mechanism, natural immunity and adaptive immunity. In natural immunity, the inborn mechanisms present in all healthy members of a species protect the body, whereas in adaptive immunity, protection is provided by alterations in the immune system induced by encounters between the immune system and specific infectious organisms. Both natural and adaptive mechanisms also come into play when the foreign substance is not infectious. Adaptive immune mechanisms operate through such components of natural immunity as phagocytic cells (found in both the blood and the tissues), eosinophilic and basophilic leukocytes (two types of blood cell), mast cells, clotting factors, and the complement system—all of which are particularly important when an allergic reaction is involved.

The principal cells of the immune system are the lymphocytes. Lymphocytes respond to foreign substances called antigens. The lymphocytes can alter their response when the same antigen is encountered again; thus they are adaptive. In subsequent encounters with an infectious antigen—for example, with measles virus—no clinically obvious reaction may be detectable. That is, a state of immunity to that particular virus has been established. On the other hand, subsequent encounters may result in an inflammatory reaction that is more intense than the original one. Poison ivy is one such response. When a reaction is harmful or is exaggerated, as in the case of poison ivy, a person is said to have a hypersensitivity reaction. Allergies are a type of hypersensitivity reaction mediated by the immune system and involving components of natural immunity. Let us now look at these components and their interaction in some detail.

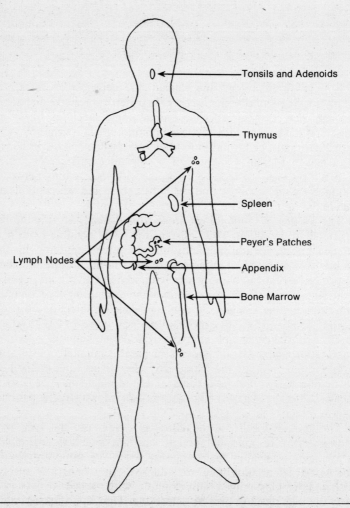

Figure 5.1.   Major Structures of the Immune System

The Immune System

Lymphocytes are derived from precursor cells called stem cells that originate in the yolk sac, liver, and bone marrow of the fetus. They circulate in the blood and lymph fluid, finally lodging in the main lymphatic organs. Bone marrow and the thymus are the primary lymphoid organs; the spleen, lymph nodes, and lymphoid masses associated with the gastrointestinal and respiratory membranes constitute the secondary, or peripheral, lymphoid organs.

Secondary lymphoid organs contain an intricate network of collagen fibers, to which phagocytic cells are attached and in which lymphocytes mix thoroughly as they move along. This process permits the lymphoid organs to act as efficient traps for foreign material that has gained access to the body. These organs are also well adapted for interaction between lymphocytes and the foreign matter.

Figure 5.2.   The Immune System—A Simplified View

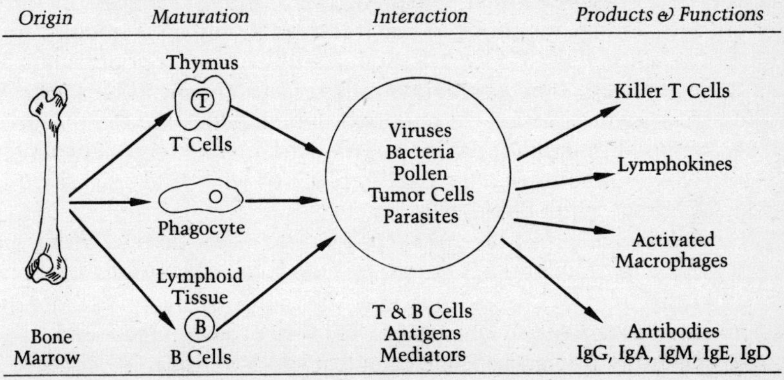

Origin	*Maturation*	*Interaction*	*Products & Functions*

The three principal types of white blood cells that participate in the immune response originate in the bone marrow.

The stem cells that remain in the bone marrow after birth are pluripotent; they continue to give rise not only to more stem cells but to all types of red and white blood cells, including lymphocytes. Moreover, they retain this ability as a person matures and becomes an adult. Those stem cells destined to become lymphocytes mature in one of two ways: they become either "T" cells or "B" cells.

During the pre- and postnatal parts of their lives, the precursors of T cells migrate from the bone marrow to the thymus (a small organ at the base of the neck), where they establish themselves and become mature T cells. For reasons that are not yet clear, as many as 90 percent of the thymic lymphocytes die within the thymus. It has been hypothesized that these are cells destined to react with "self-antigens," which, by this means, were eliminated in an attempt to avoid an autoimmune reaction. Whatever the reason, some mature T cells eventually leave the thymus and enter the body's circulatory system. In the blood, they constitute about 75 percent of the circulating lymphocytes, or about one-third of all the white blood cells in circulation. The cells can be recognized and counted by virtue of special "markers" on their surface. For example, human T cells can bind the red blood cells of a sheep to their surface. When human white blood cells are mixed with a sheep's red blood cells, the sheep's cells form small clusters around the T cells, which allows ready identification of the T cells.

In a process called cell-mediated immunity, the T cells play a major role in the body's resistance to viruses, fungi, and intracellular bacteria (for example, those that cause tuberculosis), to protozoan parasites such as those that cause African sleeping sickness, in the rejection of foreign tissue or organ transplants, and in immunity to tumors. When mature T cells are stimulated by an appropriate stimulus as an antigen, they proliferate and secrete chemical substances called lymphokines. The most important lymphokines are the macrophage migration-inhibition factor (MIF), the macrophage-activating factor (MAF), interferon, the T cell-replacing factor, and several factors that attract white blood cells.

A macrophage is a scavenger (phagocytic) cell derived from a monocyte, a particular kind of white blood cell. Macrophages are found throughout the body, but they are more likely to be found where there is chronic inflammation. They vigorously ingest and destroy numerous foreign substances and microorganisms. In contrast to T cells, which appear to respond to a limited number of antigens, macrophages ingest antigens more or less indiscriminately. In other words, it is the T cells, and not macrophages, that recognize a substance or microorganism as foreign. When a foreign substance invades the body, a group (or subset) of T cells identifies the invader and produces lymphokines, which then bring the macrophages to the site of the invasion. There the macrophages attempt to halt and destroy the foreign substance. The body's response is the same whether the substance is harmful (in the case of tuberculosis bacteria), helpful (a kidney transplant), or indifferent (poison ivy).

There are several different types of T cells in addition to those involved in cell-mediated immunity. One type, known as a cytotoxic T cell, attacks and destroys almost all foreign cells, including tumor cells, which, though not exactly foreign, differ sufficiently from normal cells for the immune system to recognize them as foreign. Two other types of T cell, "helper" T cells and "suppressor" T cells, help regulate the production of antibodies.

Lymphocytes, particularly T lymphocytes, can circulate throughout the blood and lymph and peripheral tissues, and then recirculate. They also have a lengthy life span, living as long as twenty years. Because of their circulation ability and longevity, they are superbly equipped to play a major part in the recognition and response functions of adaptive immunity.

B cells begin to mature in the bone marrow. At some point, they leave the marrow and migrate to the peripheral lymphatic tissues and organs (Figure 5.1), where they are in a good position to interact with antigens, T cells, and macrophages.

The Immune Response

Antigens are substances that induce a specific immune response. The clearest response is the appearance of antibodies in blood serum and other body fluids. The antibodies produced in this response recognize the antigen that stimulated their production; thus they can neutralize the antigen's harmful effects, if any, hastening elimination of the antigen from the body.

How is this complex sequence of events set in motion? When an antigen enters an animal, some of it is absorbed by the ever-present macrophages. The macrophages "process" the antigen, presumably enhancing the ability of some of the antigen to interact with lymphocytes. The macrophages then present the antigen to T and B cells; B cells bear a surface receptor that recognizes a specific region of the antigen, called the determinant. The B cells react with the antigen, thereby initiating an immune response. The B-cell receptor is, in fact, an antibody, the same one the B cell will eventually manufacture. Each B cell has only one type of antibody on its surface; each B cell (and its progeny, or "daughter," cells) can produce only that antibody molecule. Protein antigens may have several different determinants; this enables them to stimulate many different B cells to divide, to differentiate, and to generate clones (identical daughter cells) of antibody-secreting plasma cells. Again, each cell secretes an antibody identical to the receptor on the B cell from which it was derived. Moreover, each unique antigenic determinant on an antigen can elicit antibodies that vary in their affinity (or ability to bind) and specificity (ability to recognize a particular antigen and distinguish it from the others).

The quantity and quality of antibody produced in response to a given antigen depend largely on the nature and amount of the antigen, the route it takes in the body, and the form in which it appears. In the case of pollen allergy, for example, natural exposure to the minute amounts of antigen present in inhaled pollen grains causes a significant, though still minute, amount of an antibody to be produced. This antibody is called reaginic, or IgE, antibody. In contrast, when an extract of pollen containing relatively large amounts of the same antigen is injected for treatment, relatively large amounts of an antibody that blocks the allergic reaction will be produced. We are just beginning to understand the difference between regulation of the B cells that make the reaginic antibody and regulation of the B cells that make the blocking, or IgG, antibody. For one thing, helper T cells and suppressor T cells act differently on the two groups of B cells. It is well known that genetic factors influence immune responses; for example, allergies occur more often in some families than in others. Moreover, some genes—called immune response genes—are dedicated to controlling the response to particular antigens, whereas some control the type and amount of an antibody that can be made, some the number and distribution of lymphocytes, and some the cell-surface molecules (such as transplantation antigens) involved in the recognition of antigens.

In an animal that has never encountered a particular antigen, there resides a small population of B cells committed to respond to that antigen by virtue of its specific surface receptor. When the antigen enters the body and encounters the appropriate cells, it causes these cells to divide. Some differentiate and become antibody-secreting plasma cells. The concentration of antibody in the serum rises abruptly, and the presence of this antibody increases the rate of antigen elimination. But plasma cells survive only a few weeks. As they die, the serum antibody level subsides, ending this *primary* immune response. Some B cells, however, survive as an expanded set of specifically committed, long-lived, "memory" B cells. The animal mentioned at the beginning of this paragraph is now primed for a heightened, more rapid, secondary response to the same antigen. Here we come to the explanation for the two principal characteristics of the immune response—memory and specificity. The initial encounter with an antigen leaves the animal (or human) with a greatly expanded population of lymphocytes (both T cells and B cells) that can respond when that antigen is encountered again.

Immunoglobulins

Antibodies belong to a group of proteins called immunoglobulins (abbreviated Ig) found in serum and other body fluids. An antibody is an immunoglobulin that reacts with a given antigen. For example, an Ig that binds ragweed pollen antigen is an antiragweed-pollen antibody. To understand how antibodies function, we must first understand their structure. Like all proteins, immunoglobulins are made up of smaller units called amino acids. Twenty different amino acids are found in most proteins. These amino acids are linked by peptide bonds, forming either short or long chains called, respectively, oligopeptides or polypeptides. Some proteins, including Ig molecules, consist of several polypeptide chains held together by other types of chemical bond. The polypeptide chains in a molecule usually are twisted around each other, giving the molecule the appearance of being round or ovoid. The final shape is one of the factors that determines a protein's function. This shape, in fact, is determined by the particular linear sequence of amino acids in the polypeptide chains that make up the protein molecule.

The information that determines the amino-acid sequence of every protein the body makes is encoded in the DNA (deoxyribonucleic acid) of the genes of each cell in the body. Translation of this information begins in the nucleus of a cell. The amino acids are joined together one after the other, beginning at what is called the amino terminal end of the molecule and proceeding to the carboxyl terminal end. One of the most exciting avenues of research today is the search for the mechanism that controls the sequence of amino acids in the antibody molecule. The complexity of antibody structure makes it apparent that a complex mechanism is involved.

The best-known fact about the structure of antibodies is that, in contrast to most other proteins, antibodies do not consist of a uniform set of molecules. An antibody actually is a set of molecules that differ in a number of ways but which bind to the antigen that induced their synthesis. The key to understanding the heterogeneity of an antibody was discovered in investigations of the structure of a special type of immunoglobulin called myeloma protein. Sometimes, in both humans and other animals, tumors of plasma cells, called plasmacytomas, cause a disease called multiple myeloma. Apparently, all the plasmacytoma cells in an individual suffering from multiple myeloma arise from a single plasma cell that somehow was transformed into a tumor cell. This tumor cell, along with its progeny, synthesize only one type of Ig molecule. Because the cells secrete this molecule into the serum in great abundance, it is possible for scientists to separate the myeloma immunoglobulin from a person's serum and subject it to a purification process, which continues until the serum is free of other proteins. The complete sequence of amino acids, as well as a three-dimensional structure of many of these myeloma proteins, has now been determined. Fortunately, the structure of the myeloma Ig turns out not to be different from the structure of the normal Ig—that is, the normal antibody.

From this research five major classes of immunoglobulin have been isolated: IgA, IgD, IgE, IgG, and IgM. Immunoglobulin G, present in the highest concentration in serum, has been studied the most extensively. Its structure serves as a model of the other classes of immunoglobulin. The IgG molecule shown in Figure 5.3 contains four polypeptide chains, two identical, heavy (or H) chains, and two identical, light (or L) chains. Each half of the molecule contains an H and an L chain. The chains are held together by an amino-acid bond (cysteine) on each chain. The weight of the molecule is about 160,000 daltons, one dalton being a unit of mass equal to one-sixteenth of an oxygen atom. The immunoglobulins IgD and IgE have the same four-chain structure. Serum IgA, however, may occur in the same monomeric form, or it may consist of two more units (dimer or polymer) held together by additional interchain bonds. In certain secretions—for example, tears and saliva—IgA occurs in high concentrations. Here, it consists of two basic units joined by a small polypeptide chain called a secretory piece. IgM consists of five of the basic four-chain units joined by another small polypeptide known as a J chain. Its molecular weight is about 900,000 daltons, hence the name macroglobulin.

As shown in Figure 5.3, each H or L chain is looped on itself in regions called domains, with four or five in an H chain and two in an L chain. In the IgG molecule, the first domain of each L chain lies opposite the first domain of its adjacent H chain; the same is true of the second domain of each chain. The third domain of an H chain is opposite the third domain of the other chain; this is also true of the fourth domain of each chain. Thus each IgG molecule has six pairs of overlapping domains, small globules within the larger IgG molecule.

The first domain of a chain occurs at its amino terminal end, that is, the end synthesized first. Analysis of the amino-acid sequence of

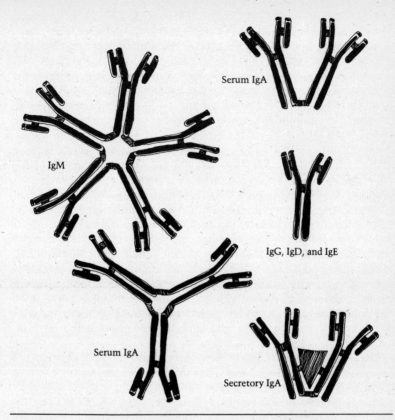

Serum IgA

IgM

IgG, IgD, and IgE

Serum IgA

Secretory IgA

Figure 5.3.   The Five Types of Antibodies

a large number of Ig molecules reveals much more sequence variability in the first 110 amino-acid positions, beginning at the amino
terminal end, of both the H and the L chains, than in the rest of the
molecule. For this reason, this part of the polypeptide chains is called
the variable (V) region. The rest of the molecule is the constant (C)
region because there is much less variability when many Ig molecules
are compared. The V and C regions of an L chain are of approximately equal length, whereas the V region comprises only 20 to 25
percent of the length of the H chain.

The heterogeneous nature of the sequence in each V region is
most evident in three or four subregions, each of which contains
ten to twelve amino acids. These regions are called hypervariable

(hv) regions. Because of the folding of the polypeptide chains in the V regions of the amino terminal H and L domains, the hv regions of each chain are extremely close to each other. In fact, they are situated in a cleftlike pocket near the amino terminal end of each half of the molecule. It is in this cleft that the antigenic determinant of an antigen molecule binds to an antibody molecule; hence, it is called the antigen-binding site of the Ig molecule. There are two identical antigen-binding sites on each IgG molecule; an IgM molecule has ten such sites. It is the particular amino acid sequence in the hv regions of a particular Ig molecule that is responsible for the unique configuration of its combining site; this configuration imparts specificity to the Ig molecule and determines its affinity for its homologous antigen. It has been estimated that a human can synthesize more than a million different combining sites, or unique antibody molecules.

Additional heterogeneity becomes apparent when the amino acid sequences of the constant regions are considered. These regions (about one hundred residues long in the L chain and three hundred to four hundred residues long in the H chain) are only relatively constant when different molecules are compared. Nevertheless, except for small differences due to genetic polymorphisms, it is possible to place the C-region sequences in a small number of major groups, two for the L chain (kappa and lambda) and five for the H chain (alpha, delta, epsilon, gamma, and mu).

These differences in H-chain sequence are what distinguish the five classes of immunoglobulin. The differences in sequence are also responsible for differences in the function of the major classes of immunoglobulin. For example, IgE is the immunoglobulin responsible for allergic reactions. Within these classes, smaller variations in C-region sequences define Ig subclasses. For instance, there are four subclasses of IgG in humans: IgG1, IgG2, IgG3, and IgG4. To a certain extent, these subclasses differ in their properties. Because no subclasses of IgE have been identified thus far, researchers believe that all IgE molecules have an equal effect in mediating an allergic reaction.

Also of interest are the patterns of Ig classes that occur in various immune responses. Usually, IgM antibodies predominate in a primary immune response. In most secondary responses, IgG antibodies predominate, but smaller amounts of IgA and IgM antibodies are also produced. Some infectious diseases cause antibodies—mainly IgM—to be produced, whereas other diseases induce the production primarily of IgG antibodies. IgA antibodies predominate in most external secretions. IgD antibodies are located on the surface of B lymphocytes; very little ever appears in serum. The production of

IgE antibodies seems to be favored when the antigen dose is extremely small, when the dose is absorbed via the respiratory or gastrointestinal tract, or when, in experiments with animals, it is injected after adsorption on alum.

To recapitulate, antibody is produced by sets of lymphocytes in response to a specific stimulus, or antigen. Antibodies are capable of binding the antigens that induced the formation of the antibodies. An antibody, in fact, is a collection of different protein molecules, all of which can bind the same antigen. All antibodies belong to the group of serum proteins called immunoglobulins. Only when an immunoglobulin is known to bind a particular antigen is it referred to as an antibody against that antigen, and only a small proportion of the total immunoglobulin in serum can be associated with specific antibody activity; the remainder must be regarded as nonspecific, although antigens probably exist with which it will react.

There are five major classes of immunoglobulin. An antibody against a given antigen usually contains immunoglobulins that belong to more than one of the five classes, and various antibody pools contain different proportions of each immunoglobulin. An antibody of each class has a different set of functions. The principal function of most antibodies is to resist infection; antibodies, however, may also be involved in a pathological reaction—for example, in an allergy.

Immunopathologic Reactions

For simplicity, pathological reactions with an immunologic basis are grouped according to four types, I through IV.

Type I—immediate hypersensitivity. An immediate hypersensitivity (anaphylactic) reaction is mediated by the IgE antibody on mast cells and basophil leukocytes. An antigen interacting with cell-bound IgE antibodies causes the release of a group of substances known as mediators. These substances are most directly responsible for the major clinical manifestations of immediate hypersensitivity, the symptoms of which usually begin within minutes after exposure to an antigen. When this type of reaction occurs in humans, it is called an allergic reaction, or allergy. Hay fever, some forms of asthma and hives (urticaria), anaphylactic shock, and some reactions that occur after insect stings or the ingestion of certain drugs or foods are examples of IgE-mediated hypersensitivity reactions. It is well known that clinical manifestations of IgE-mediated reactions may persist for hours, days, or even weeks. When this occurs, additional pathological mechanisms must be invoked.

Type II—cytotoxic reactions. Cytotoxic reactions are those in which an IgG antibody directed against a cell membrane component reacts with the component and, in so doing, activates the body's complement system. The complement system consists of interacting proteins (some of which are enzymes) in series which, when activated, react in a cascade manner. The end product of this reaction is the destruction of the membrane of the cells or the bacteria. The untoward reaction following a transfusion of incompatible blood is one example of an IgG antibody-mediated cytotoxic reaction.

Type III—immune complexes. Type III reactions are those in which immune complexes form. That is, aggregates containing many molecules of antigen and antibody, mainly of the IgG and IgM classes, are formed. Immune complexes can become localized in small blood vessels, where they activate the complement system, producing local, acute inflammation. When an antigen is injected into the skin of a sensitized animal, an area of local swelling and erythema appears

Figure 5.4. Pathways of Complement Activation

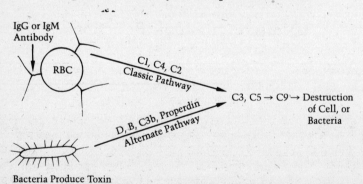

The complement system consists of a series of interacting enzymes which can be activated in either of two ways. In one, known as the classical pathway, the system is turned on when antibody reacts with an antigen such as a red blood cell (RBC), forming an immune complex. This complex binds C1, the first enzyme in the series, and the cascade reaction begins. In the alternate pathway, certain substances—such as the toxins (poisons) produced by bacteria—trigger the latter part of the cascade.

Table 5.1. Allergic Reactions

TYPE AND NUMBER		MECHANISM	EXAMPLES
Type I	Immediate hypersensitivity or anaphylactic	IgE antibody on mast cell reacts with antigen resulting in release of mediators	Hay fever; allergic reaction to insect sting; allergic shock
Type II	Cytotoxic	IgG antibody reacts with cell membranes or antigen associated with cell membrane	Transfusion of incompatible blood types
Type III	Arthus	Antigen and antibody bind together to form immune complexes which deposit in walls of blood vessels or kidneys	Serum sickness; some drug reactions
Type IV	Delayed hypersensitivity or cell-mediated	T cells interact directly with antigen	Poison ivy; graft rejection

after one to two hours. This condition will peak in three to six hours; after that, it usually subsides. This is known as the Arthus reaction. Serum sickness is a more generalized immunopathology (vasculitis) caused by circulating immune complexes. Some reactions to drugs are mediated by the immune-complex mechanism.

Type IV—delayed hypersensitivity. The tuberculin test is the classic example of a type IV reaction. In this type, a local reaction occurs in the skin twenty-four to forty-eight hours after injection of tuberculin in a person sensitive to tuberculin. This reaction is also known as a cell-mediated immune response. Sensitized T cells interact with antigen, proliferate, then secrete substances called lymphokines. Lymphokines draw other cells, principally monocytes, from the blood to the site of the antigen. The local reaction, then, results from the interaction of monocytes (which are transformed into macrophages) with the localized deposit of antigen. This reaction can produce immunity in the case of an infectious agent, such as Mycobacterium, the cause of tuberculosis. Rejection of tissue or an organ transplant from one individual to another is also an example of cell-mediated reaction.

Mechanisms of Allergic Reactions

The most common hypersensitivity reaction is the allergic reaction. In susceptible people, IgE antibodies are induced when an individual is exposed to such antigens as airborne pollen of grasses, trees, or weeds; animal dander, urine, or saliva; mold spores; various insect-derived dusts and airborne, organic dusts; the venom of stinging insects; or certain drugs and foods. Allergens are antigens that produce allergic reactions. As encountered in nature, most allergenic substances contain many different antigens, that is, molecules capable of inducing an immune response. Most of the time, however, only a few of the antigens in these substances act as allergens. In recent years, allergens from a few pollen and animal sources have been identified, characterized, and, in some instances, isolated in pure form. So far, these allergens have proved to be proteins, mostly those in the molecular weight range of 10,000 to 40,000 daltons but which otherwise have no special chemical features.

Most commercially available allergenic products used in diagnosis and therapy are simple aqueous extracts of one or more source materials, such as pollen or animal dander. The biologically active components in these extracts comprise only a small proportion of the total number of components in the extracts. Further, only a few allergenic products have been standardized with respect to their active ingredients. Application of the methods of modern biochemistry and immunology to the analysis of allergenic extracts, however, should result in rapid improvement of the quality of the products available to physicians.

We do not yet know what it is that leads to the spontaneous production of large amounts of IgE antibodies in some people. Recent evidence suggests that a person's total IgE level is genetically determined—perhaps by a single gene. The normal, adult IgE level is less than 750 nanograms (abbreviated ng; 1 nanogram is less than 1 billionth of an ounce) per milliliter (about 350 International units per milliliter), with a mean of 100 to 200 ng/ml (50 to 100 I.u./ml). In allergic individuals, this level is often two to four times above normal, presumably as a result of the individual's immune response to environmental allergens. In people infected with certain common parasitic worms, the total serum IgE may be as high as 200,000 ng/ml; usually, however, only a small proportion of this total is parasite-specific IgE antibody. Although the latter finding is thought to indicate that IgE antibodies play a role in immunity to these parasites, there is still no compelling evidence to confirm this hypothesis.

As we saw above, exposure to small doses of antigen tends to favor IgE antibody production, production that is regulated by both helper and suppressor T cells. Scientists now know that the level of IgE antibody specific for ragweed-pollen antigens rises dramatically during and immediately after the annual ragweed-pollen season. The level then falls slowly until the next pollen season, when it again rises. It appears that the annual boost in the production of specific IgE antibody keeps the level of IgE antibody sufficiently high to produce symptoms in individuals exposed to large enough amounts of allergen. Interestingly, even though a pollen-sensitive individual may be exposed to allergen for only a few weeks over a year, this person continues to synthesize enough IgE antibody to maintain detectable serum and tissue levels throughout the year. It has been suggested, but not proved, that this may result from a disturbance among regulatory T cells in people who produce enough IgE to make them allergic.

Measuring IgE

The measurement of serum IgE levels, first made possible by the discovery in 1967 of a patient with IgE myeloma, is of interest to physicians because elevations in serum IgE levels occur more frequently in allergic individuals. The reader should remember, though, that the total serum IgE measurement is not a specific diagnostic test for allergy.

Subsequent purification of IgE, and the preparation of antibody specific for human IgE (anti-IgE), led to the development of laboratory procedures for measuring total IgE and allergen-specific IgE. These new diagnostic methods supplement the traditional skin test, which gives only partially complete quantitative information about specific IgE antibody.

Several methods, called radioimmunoassay methods, are now available for measuring total serum IgE. The competitive radioimmunosorbent test (RIST) is a competitive-binding assay in which IgE in the test sample competes with IgE that has been tagged with radioactive iodine. In this test, the IgE content of the serum is inversely proportional to the radioactivity bound by the anti-IgE. The absolute level of IgE is obtained by comparing it with a standard curve derived from a serum containing a known amount of IgE. The RIST method has limited sensitivity, however, primarily because of the variability among samples containing less than 100 nanograms of IgE per milliliter.

In the noncompetitive RIST method, a sample of test serum is incubated with solid-phase anti-IgE in the absence of labeled IgE. The solid-phase anti-IgE is then washed and incubated with anti-IgE labeled with radioactive iodine, which, in turn, binds to the IgE on the solid phase. The radioactivity binds in proportion to the amount of IgE bound during the first incubation, and is directly proportional to the IgE content of the serum sample. Because of improvements in sensitivity and precision, this procedure is now the method of choice for measuring serum IgE.

Of perhaps greater interest is the measurement of specific IgE antibody using the radioallergosorbent test (RAST). This test is similar to the noncompetitive RIST, except that allergen, rather than anti-IgE, is bound to the solid-phase matrix. After incubation of solid-phase allergen (allergosorbent) with serum, the matrix is washed and then incubated with labeled anti-IgE. The amount of radioactivity that binds to the allergosorbent is directly proportional to the allergen-specific IgE antibody in the serum sample. The result is expressed as "antibody titer" relative to that of a designated reference serum. Recent modifications of the RAST method permit quantification of absolute amounts of IgE antibody specific for several purified allergens. But interpretation of the results is still uncertain, especially when the values obtained are not highly elevated because of a fairly wide overlap of nonallergic and allergic individuals in the lower range of values. RAST, therefore, is still mainly a semiquantitative, diagnostic screening procedure. The more sensitive skin test still has greater diagnostic significance, particularly when the test results are borderline.

Two types of cell must be considered in discussing allergic reactions: mast cells and basophil leukocytes. Mast cells, located near the small blood vessels, are found in connective tissue throughout the body. This is clearly a convenient location for cells associated with the functioning of the blood vessels. We do not yet know exactly where mast cells originate, although evidence recently uncovered suggests that some mast cells come from the bone marrow, while others are derived from lymphocytes. If we are to understand the role of mast cells in allergic reactions, we must learn more about their origin. One thing we do know is that mast cells are long-lived, though just how long is uncertain.

Basophil leukocytes are the progeny of the same stem cells (located in the bone marrow) that produce such other types of white blood cell as neutrophils and eosinophils. As basophils mature (perhaps under the influence of T cells), they leave the bone marrow and enter the blood, where they appear to remain for only one or two days. Then the basophils leave the blood and enter the extravascular spaces, most often at sites of allergic reactions or where parasites have lodged. Many apparently exit the body by moving into the respiratory or the gastrointestinal tract.

Both mast cells and basophils have an abundance of dense granules in their cytoplasm. These cells can be identified in the light microscope only when the granules are specially stained. Each granule is surrounded by a membrane that effectively insulates the contents of the granule from the rest of the cell. Granules contain a high concentration of histamine, which is held there because it is bound to the anticoagulant heparin and to a protein matrix.

IgE molecules have a rather high affinity for the surface of mast cells and basophils. This affinity is due to the presence of molecules (receptors) on the cell's surface, which recognize certain unique structural features of the constant region of the IgE molecule. In both normal and allergic people, IgE molecules are bound to mast cells and basophils. In allergic individuals, however, some of these molecules are antibody molecules specific to one or more allergens. Thus the cells in an allergic person are said to be sensitized; when allergen reaches them, they respond characteristically.

An allergic reaction is said to begin when an allergen molecule interacts with two specific IgE antibody molecules on the surface of a sensitized mast cell or a basophil. Exactly how the bridging of two antibody molecules by an allergen induces the cell to respond is still not known. What is known is that the cell can be triggered in the absence of either antigen or antibody. All that must be done is to bridge two of the surface receptor molecules; this is true even when IgE is not present. The triggering process has recently been accomplished with antibody specific for the mast cell receptor itself. A number of biochemical changes have been detected in mast cells and basophils immediately after they are triggered by the interaction of allergen with IgE antibody. The change most thoroughly studied occurs in the cyclic nucleotide system, in which the cyclic adenosine monophosphate (cAMP) concentration falls, while that of the cyclic guanosine monophosphate (cGMP) rises. A fall in the cAMP-cGMP

Figure 5.5. IgE Antibodies

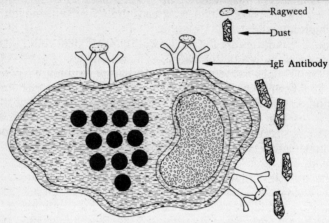

Each IgE antibody will react only with the allergen against which it was made. This means that an IgE antibody made against a ragweed pollen will only react with another grain of ragweed pollen. This is why it is important to know those substances to which one is allergic. When an allergic person again encounters this allergen, it binds to the IgE antibodies that are already sitting on the surface of the mast cells or basophils.

Figure 5.6. Combination of Allergen and Antibody

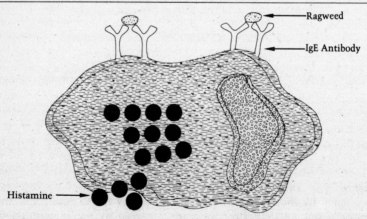

This combination of allergen and antibody is a signal to the mast cells and basophils to release the little packets of chemicals that they contain, including histamine. These powerful chemicals or mediators, as they are known, can then cause various symptoms of allergy, such as wheezing, sneezing, runny eyes, itching, abdominal pain, retching or diarrhea.

ratio favors the entry of calcium ions into the cell. In a process called degranulation, an increase in the concentration of intracellular calcium leads immediately to secretion of the contents of the granule from the cell into the surrounding body fluid. This process, however, does not result in destruction of the cell. Degranulation operates thus: triggering of the cell causes the cell's surface membrane to move up against the membrane surrounding the granules (which are just beneath the surface). The two membranes quickly fuse, and an opening forms at the site. As the opening enlarges, the interior of the granule is exposed to the fluid outside the cell. The contents of the granule are now effectively outside the cell. Note that the membrane of the cell remains intact, with the membrane of the granule now incorporated in it. At this point, the histamine quickly dissolves out of the granule and diffuses into the surrounding tissue. There it acts directly on adjacent small blood vessels, making them leaky to the fluid of the blood. This, in turn, leads to edema, or swelling of the tissues, and acts on the nerve endings, causing an itching sensation. When this happens in the skin, it is called hives. The process is the same that occurs when a doctor performs a skin test on an allergic patient, using a dilute solution of allergenic extract. A local reaction appears within a few minutes, then fades within twenty to thirty minutes. This is an immediate hypersensitivity reaction.

Histamine also acts on smooth, or nonskeletal, muscle—for example, on the tiny muscles in the bronchial tree—causing them to contract and making the air passages in the lungs narrower. This condition is called bronchospasm, or asthma. Histamine can also act on mucous glands, causing the secretion of thin, watery mucus—a condition that usually occurs in the noses of allergic people during the hay fever season.

Histamine is only one of the "mediators" of anaphylaxis released when mast cells or basophils are triggered by the interaction of allergens and IgE. Other substances that are released, for which there is evidence of a role in allergic inflammation, are:

1. SRS-A, a slow-reaction substance of anaphylaxis, known as leukotriene, that was recently identified as a product of arachidonic acid metabolism. It acts on smooth muscles.

2. ECF-A, an eosinophil chemotactic factor of anaphylaxis that consists of several different short peptide chains. It acts as an attractant to eosinophils.

3. PAF, a factor recently identified as an acetyl glycerylether compound. It activates platelets, small blood corpuscles that contain additional mediators, and anticoagulants.

Figure 5.7.   Mediators Released from Human Mast Cells and Basophils

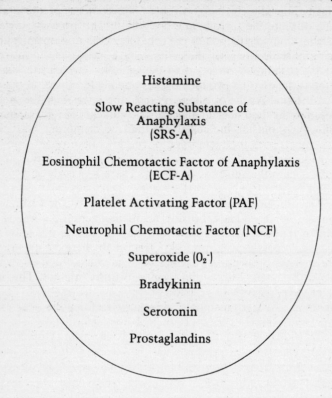

Histamine

Slow Reacting Substance of
Anaphylaxis
(SRS-A)

Eosinophil Chemotactic Factor of Anaphylaxis
(ECF-A)

Platelet Activating Factor (PAF)

Neutrophil Chemotactic Factor (NCF)

Superoxide (O_2^-)

Bradykinin

Serotonin

Prostaglandins

Other mediators (see Figure 5.7) may be involved in allergic reactions, but their role is unclear.

The explosive release of mediators from mast cells and basophils depends on where the reaction occurs. Most allergic reactions occur in the eyes, nose and throat, lungs, intestines, or skin. In a condition known as anaphylactic shock, the entire body is affected. The intensity of an allergic reaction depends somewhat on the concentration of mediators that reach their targets in the tissues and on how long-acting they are. Powerful inactivators of each mediator occur in the blood and the tissues, limiting this concentration and duration. To a certain degree, the intensity and duration of a particular allergic reaction depend on the number of mast cells and basophils in the tissues at the time of the allergen-IgE antibody interaction. Their number is not constant in the target tissues. During the ragweed-pollen season, for example, mast cells and basophils appear in greater numbers in the membrane that lines the nasal cavity, as well as in the abundant mucus typical of hay fever. When these cells are concentrated in the nose, much more mediator exists to be released after pollen is inhaled. This condition may have something to do with the fact that symptoms of ragweed hay fever can continue for days or weeks after the actual ragweed pollen season has ended. We do not know exactly what causes the influx of these cells during the pollen season, or what accounts for their disappearance after the season. It will not be surprising, though, if it turns out that T cells have something to do with the influx of mast cells and basophils.

Figure 5.8.   Allergic Reaction and IgG Antibodies Blocking Reaction

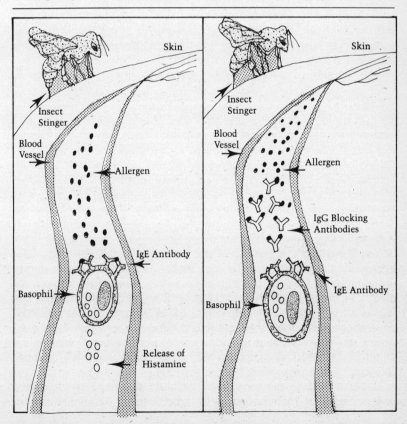

Treating Allergic Diseases

Drugs commonly used to treat allergic diseases act either by suppressing the release of mediators from mast cells and basophils (disodium cromoglycate acts in this way) or by antagonizing the effect of the mediators on tissue targets (antihistamines). The action mechanism of corticosteroids such as prednisone is not known. Recent evidence suggests that corticosteroids may reduce the number of mast cells and basophils in the target tissues. As more is learned about allergic reactions and how mediators act, improved drugs can be developed.

The simplest, most straightforward way to relieve the symptoms of allergic diseases is to avoid the allergens that cause them. This is done fairly easily when the source of the allergen can be recognized and avoided, as, for example, in the case of a pet cat. When the source is as widespread as ragweed pollen, however, avoidance is not practical.

In this century, extracts containing biologically active components of allergens have been used extensively in treating allergic diseases. At first, immunotherapy, the regular, systematic administration of these extracts, was intended to immunize people against the supposed toxic effect of allergens. As the role of hypersensitivity in allergic diseases became known, the concept of hyposensitization was introduced, in which successful immunotherapy was thought to result in a reduced level of sensitivity. But it did not result in a complete loss of sensitivity. Later it was shown that immunotherapy induces a new type of antibody, called a blocking antibody. The use of modern immunologic methods has proved that the blocking antibody is an IgG antibody capable of reacting with allergen in the body fluids before it reaches the mast cells and basophils in target organs. Elevation of allergen-specific IgG antibody does indeed occur during immunotherapy; this seems important in the successful treatment of allergy to stinging insects. It has also been found that immunotherapy blunts the seasonal booster effect of inhaled allergen on IgE antibody. This effect is followed by a gradual decline in the level of the particular antibody. What is not yet clear is whether these changes account for the relief of symptoms that occurs with successful immunotherapy for allergy to such inhaled substances as pollen.

Another clue to the mechanism of immunotherapy is the recent observation that immunotherapy is accompanied by an increase in suppressor T cells. It seems reasonable to assume that these T cells are related to the changes described above. Furthermore, it is possible that the T cells are also involved in regulating the flow of basophils and mast cells to target organs. If such is the case, perhaps another effect of immunotherapy will be a reduction in the number of sensitized cells present in the target tissues of an individual being treated. Further research in the immunologic aspects of allergic diseases should provide a better understanding of their mechanisms and should, as well, put immunotherapy on a more rational basis.

Summary

The term *allergy* (derived from *antigen*, a substance capable of giving rise to the production of antibody) was coined by Baron Clemens von Pirquet in 1906 to indicate a state of changed reaction to a foreign substance (which von Pirquet called an *allergen*). Allergens, von Pirquet said, differ from antigens, in that they can lead not to the production of antibody but to a condition of hypersensitivity. In his view, the term *immunity* should be restricted to those processes in which the introduction of a foreign substance into an individual does not cause a reaction that can be detected with medical tests; in such cases, individuals would be in a state of complete insensitivity.

On that basis, it is apparent that, to understand and control allergic diseases, we must understand the immune system. In this century we have seen a remarkable expansion of our knowledge of the immune system, knowledge that has been used to gain insight into the relationship of the immune system to allergic diseases. Further advances in the ability to diagnose and treat allergic diseases depends largely on the application of this knowledge to the treatment of allergic people.

Author's Note

Because the field of immunology is so broad, this chapter could only highlight a few of its salient features. For a comprehensive treatment of the field of immunology, the interested reader is referred to: Samter, *Immunological Diseases*, 2nd ed. (Boston: Little, Brown, 1971); Middleton et al., *Allergy Principles and Practice* (Saint Louis: C. V. Mosby, 1978); and Fudenberg et al., *Basic and Clinical Immunology* (Los Altos, Cal.: Lange Medical Publications, 1980).

CHAPTER 6

Allergy Research
by Gail G. Shapiro, M.D.

An allergy is a reaction, usually between antibodies, or specific proteins, manufactured by the body of an allergic person and foreign proteins inhaled or ingested by that person. The result is a release of allergic mediators, humoral substances produced by the body that are capable of causing such undesirable effects as itching, redness, runny nose, and wheezing. Sometimes, instead of causing the release of chemical mediators, the foreign substances that are present produce a reaction of lymphocytes and macrophages—a cellular rather than a humoral response.

Any attempt to understand allergic reactions raises numerous important questions. What makes someone "allergic," that is, capable of reacting to inhaled or ingested proteins, or both, in a potentially dangerous way, whereas someone else has no reaction at all? How is this allergic potential passed from generation to generation? How is a person's ability to be allergic modulated? Can this potential be controlled? How does this allergic potential change as people change? Can they "grow into" or "out of" allergies, and can they influence whether they do this by what they eat and breathe?

The answers to these questions have much to do with whether a person is allergic. But just as many questions remain about specific allergic conditions. For example, why do some people have rashes while others have hay fever, and still others, asthma? Why do young children often develop eczema first and then rhinitis, finally becoming asthmatic? Is medical science capable of halting the progression from one allergic problem to another? What is different about an allergic person who experiences only hay fever, and one who suffers from asthma? Why are an asthmatic's lungs sensitive to environmental stimuli, while the sensitivity of the sufferer from hay fever is confined to the nose? What about the drugs that are now used for allergic disease? Do we know the optimal doses of drugs for skin rashes, rhinitis, and asthma? How do physicians go about weighing drug risks against benefits? What is the theoretical basis for the many pharmacologic agents used today?

Types of Allergy Research

What about treatment in the future? What techniques do scientists use to develop new methods of treatment? How can they be certain of the safety of a treatment for humans? What are the requirements of proper research? What constraints are placed on research, constraints that sometimes delay the marketing of new drugs?

All these questions are relevant to allergy research. Both patients and physicians needs to be better informed about this research, which involves population studies, laboratory studies, experiments using animals, and finally, testing in humans.

Epidemiological Research

Some scientists specialize in research on the inheritance of allergy characteristics. They study people, examining traits and how these people pass the traits on to their children. They study such characteristics as the presence of asthma and allergic rhinitis, or eczema, trying to establish the frequency with which these diseases appear in succeeding generations.

Basic Laboratory

Some researchers approach allergies from a different direction; they spend years in the laboratory studying the cells involved in allergic reactions. Others try to understand how the cells work. Still others go on to discover how the behavior of these cells changes. Some researchers study the chemicals that are released during an allergic reaction; others attempt to modify the release of these chemicals by changing the environment.

Animal

Much of the research today consists of studies of allergies in animals. Because certain species develop allergic sensitivity to specific chemicals, they can be used to study the process of allergic sensitization. Research in animals can also be used to develop new methods of desensitization. Animals are necessary in tests of new drugs, since all new pharmacologic agents must somehow be proven safe before they can be tested in humans.

Human

Research in humans takes several different avenues. A major area involves the observation of normal body functions and determination of which ranges are to be considered normal and which are deviations. A great many people must be studied under a variety of conditions before researchers can determine what is normal and what is not among people subjected to various changes in their environments.

Once the definition of what is normal has been established, the next step involves observing and comparing differences between normally functioning people and those who are suffering from specific abnormalities. Another major area concerns the pharmacologic modification of disease states—how drugs affect the way people function, as well as how the drugs can be used to improve people's health.

In short, human investigation is a heterogenous subject encompassing the definition of normal function, observation comparing normal and abnormal functions, elucidation of the way environmental factors affect people, and investigation of how pharmacologic agents modify physiology.

Safeguards in Human Research The description and pharmacologic modification of disease are of paramount interest to everyone involved—clinical practitioners, scientists, and patients alike. We must not, however, allow the fight against disease to lead to abuse of human volunteers or to the development of potentially harmful remedies produced for large-scale consumption. Protecting human volunteers is, or should be, the concern of all researchers. Volunteers deserve a thorough explanation of the risks and possible consequences of research.

To ensure that subjects receive proper treatment, most research centers have a "human-subject review committee" composed of physicians and lay individuals who judge prospective research projects to determine whether the projects are safe for humans and whether they are appropriate for human participation. These committees make sure that research is explained to volunteers—both verbally and in writing—and that both written and verbal consent are obtained before a person participates in a scientific study. Most review committees assess projects on a continuing basis. In general, universities and research institutions do not sanction research in humans that does not meet the standards of the committee involved. Similarly, reputable scientific journals have policies of not publishing the results of experimentation in humans unless the research has been reviewed and approved.

One aspect of the research review process is that of new drugs. Although new drugs offer the possibility of solving old problems, they also pose serious threats if not adequately evaluated ahead of time. The U.S. Food and Drug Administration (FDA) is charged with investigating and licensing drugs in the United States, which involves the strict regulation of tests of new products and clinical investigators. Usually, the investigators are physicians who wish to use volunteers in clinical trials of new drugs not yet approved.

To be approved, a new drug must undergo several phases of investigation. The first phase is that of experiments in animals. In this phase, laboratory animals are studied so that obvious toxicity can be ruled out. If a drug passes this stage successfully, it is cleared for the first phase of human research and is administered to a small number of normal human volunteers. This part of the testing is designed to ascertain a drug's safety before its use for specific diseases. From this phase the drug moves to phase 2 of the investigation, where it is studied in a few human subjects with health problems which, it is believed, the drug under investigation will relieve. The drug is tested for safety and effectiveness at specific dosage levels. Information about the best dosage and frequency of administration is often determined in this phase of research. The next phase, phase 3, involves testing on a greater scale, to gain information about the effectiveness and possible side effects of the drug under study. The final phase, phase 4, is conducted after the drug has been marketed, and involves large-scale, long-term testing of the drug. It is easy to understand why many years may pass before all phases of the testing of a new drug have been completed to everyone's satisfaction, both the FDA's and the manufacturer's. This period is often frustrating for patients and physicians, but it is essential if mistakes with potentially dangerous consequences, are to be avoided.

The Organization of Research

Before any allergy problem is solved, or any theory of allergy is tested, certain fundamental criteria must be satisfied. A patient who receives a drug may not be aware of the planning and thought that went into the research leading to approval of the drug or drugs the patient uses and depends on every day.

The question to be answered in the research must first be identified clearly. Then time and effort must be devoted to organizing the research. For example, how many subjects should be used? How many comparison groups? How many observations, and what type, should be made? What should be the duration of observations for the observations to be meaningful? For comparisons to be statistically significant, the volunteers must be allocated without bias to treatment groups. Researchers are constantly concerned about how data is collected so that results will be unbiased and valid.

It is no wonder that researchers become upset when unsubstantiated, sensational statements are made claiming, for instance, breakthroughs in research. Unless hypotheses and breakthroughs in therapy are confirmed by scientific tests and properly designed experimentation, they do not deserve public acceptance and confidence.

In reviewing research in the field of allergy, both current and future, researchers often start with population studies that have been used to gain information about the characteristics of an allergic disease and the frequency with which it occurs.

Epidemiologic and Basic Laboratory Research

We now take an overview of knowledge recently acquired through research, and glance at projects for the near future. We will discuss population studies, basic laboratory work, and human research in specific allergic conditions.

Epidemiologic

Population studies reveal that 17 percent of the American people are affected by at least one allergic disease. Approximately 5 percent of American children suffer from asthma. Although allergic disease does not prevail in any particular socioeconomic class, it does affect some families more than others. Inheritance definitely plays a role in the occurrence of asthma and allergic rhinitis among close relatives of some family members; the specific characteristics of inheritance, however, are as yet poorly understood. Also, people with one allergic disease are more likely than the general population to have other allergic conditions.

The cost of allergic disease in the United States exceeds $1 billion a year. This figure includes physicians' fees, hospital care and medications, and such indirect costs as earnings lost because of time away from work. Asthma is one of the leading causes of visits to physicians. Meanwhile, it has been shown that outpatient care by allergists significantly reduces both the incidence and the duration of inpatient care, or hospital stays. Allergic disease is also a major cause of friction in families. An asthmatic child who suffers from frequent episodes of bronchospasm at night may disturb the family's sleep while arousing the worry and fears of the child's parents and brothers and sisters.

Much more information is needed concerning environmental influences on allergic disease. Although scientific knowledge of the influence of environment on people with asthma is incomplete, scientists do know that even normal individuals suffer from smaller air passages caused by exposure to smoke. This suggests that asthmatics suffer even more from such exposure.

The influence of inheritance in allergic disease needs to be better understood, in addition to gaining a better understanding of the interaction of environment and inheritance. More large-scale population studies, in which groups of Americans in varying geographic and socioeconomic settings are observed, should help.

Basic Laboratory

Allergic disease occurs when the body mounts a specific response to foreign substances in the environment. A vast amount of research has been devoted to understanding the foreign substances, or antigens, that initiate these responses and the many ways in which the body reacts to the antigens.

Most antigens are complex molecules. Because of their dissimilarity to the body's natural proteins, the body can recognize them as foreign. These antigens are usually made up of specific, recognizable determinants bound to a carrier substance. Specific determinants stimulate certain cells (B lymphocytes) of the immune system, producing antibodies directed against the determinants. The carrier molecules stimulate T lymphocytes, which may be helpers or suppressors of the B lymphocytes' productivity. Both B and T cells cooperate in producing an antibody response to foreign proteins.

During the 1970s, an extensive study was made of the immune response mechanism. The two major classes of lymphocytes—B and T—were distinguished and separated on the basis of different surface characteristics. Modulation of the cells that produce antibodies is of major importance. B lymphocytes differentiate into plasma cells that produce antibodies, proteins with determinants capable of recognizing antigens and that result from immune mechanisms. The classes of immunoglobulin are IgA, IgD, IgE, IgG, and IgM. Immunoglobulins are composed of molecules held together in a specific array. Portions of these molecules recognize and react with foreign proteins (antigens), whereas other portions attach to and react with cells and biologically active molecules of the body. The interaction of antigen and immunoglobulin then results in immune responses and/or allergic manifestations in an individual.

Immunoglobulin E is the antibody most frequently associated with allergic disease. It is bound to cells in the respiratory tract, gastrointestinal tract, and skin. After it has been formed by initial exposure and response to an antigen, a subsequent antigen challenge produces an interaction that results in the release of mediators capable of causing such allergic manifestations as wheezing or runny nose, depending on the level of exposure and the individual's reaction pattern. Research in the future will likely be aimed at refining knowledge of antigen molecules, identifying those that can be used in allergy testing and the study of immune response mechanisms.

The recognition and description of T lymphocytes has recently advanced to a sophisticated level. These cells serve at least four distinct functions. First, "helper" T cells appear to energize B cells and make it easier for them to produce immunoglobulins. They are stimulated when antigens are processed by macrophages, a type of cell. The macrophage-processed antigen stimulates T helper cells, which stimulate the production of B cells. Second, T cells kill other cells in a process called cytolysis. In addition to their ability to kill, cytotoxic T cells play a major role in rejecting such foreign cells as transplanted tissues, tumors, and viruses. The third function of the T cell is production of lymphokines, chemicals that regulate immune events, for example, the migration of cells to sites of immune reactivity. Fourth, suppressor T cells prevent B cells from producing antibody. Current research suggests that allergic immunotherapy helps suppress allergic symptoms by stimulating suppressor T cells, which, in turn, prevent allergic antibody IgE from being produced in the usual amounts.

Investigators in basic research have begun to isolate some of the factors involved in the inheritance of allergic tendencies. Largely through experiments in which animals with known genetic makeups were inbred and their immune responses were evaluated, it has been observed that certain genes control the function of T cells and thereby determine an individual's immune response to a particular stimulus.

Thus immune reactivity is programmed as part of an individual's genetic structure. The amount of IgE a person has may be controlled by a single IgE regulator gene, which depends on T cells to carry out its instructions.

Research has shown that, in addition to antigen recognition and antibody production, numerous other biological systems contribute to the versatility and complexity of the immune response. Considerable research effort continues to be devoted to characterizing the numerous interactions.

Asthma

While much creative energy is being devoted to basic research in the mechanisms that underlie the immune response, other allergic disease entities are being studied. We now shift our focus from the laboratory to an examination of some specific diseases currently being studied.

Although asthma is usually defined as a reversible obstruction of the air passages, knowledge of the structural changes that occur in asthma has been gained through examination of the lungs of people who have died of severe, nonreversible asthma. An asthmatic tends to have overly reactive, smooth muscles in the bronchial tree. Muscle constriction, increased mucous secretion, and swelling of the lining of the air passages all contribute to attacks. Secretions occasionally become so thick that obstruction is complete and fatal.

The air passages, or airways, are controlled to some extent by nervous innervation, in which the signals for muscle relaxation and those for constriction are unbalanced. The nervous system itself, or the receptors of the signals to the bronchial tree, or both, may be faulty in individuals with asthma. Understanding the possible defect in control mechanisms involves vigorous research. The term *nervous*, as used in this context, does not imply psychological or psychosomatic involvement but rather refers to the autonomic nervous system which controls involuntary processes. The effect a person's psychological makeup has on asthma is a subject for later discussion.

During an asthma attack, special chemicals called mediators are released into lung tissue and the circulatory system that promote constriction of the smooth muscles, secretion of mucus, and swelling of tissue. Scientists are expanding the knowledge of these mediators— where they are produced, what effect they have, and how that effect is achieved. Another aspect of this research concerns the mechanisms involved in quelling asthma attacks by inactivating or modifying the mediators.

The first step in searching for the optimal therapy is observation of the changes that occur in asthma. Medication that helps relax bronchial muscles or that halts the release of an allergic mediator is discussed in other chapters. Much research effort has been devoted to study of the chemistry of these drugs, with an eye to improving their therapeutic properties while diminishing side effects. Another aspect of research in therapeutics is the leap from the laboratory, where the structure and function of a drug are first observed, to clinical situations, where the reactions of volunteers are evaluated in ascertaining the drug's safety and effectiveness. Other research focuses on measuring the active drug in the body fluids in an attempt to determine optimal dosages.

In summary, asthma research efforts are aimed at delineating the pathological changes that occur during and after an asthma attack and a better understanding of the pharmacologic modification of the problem.

Allergic Rhinitis

Rhinitis is inflammation of the nose. Allergic rhinitis occurs when an individual who is allergic to a foreign antigen, and who has antibodies against the antigen (bound to mast cells of the nasal mucosa), inhales the antigen. When antigen and tissue-bound antibody interreact, mediators are released by the mast cells. These mediators cause dilatation of the blood vessels, leakage of fluid, and swelling of membranes, as well as increased production of mucus. Recent work has led to a clearer understanding of the mechanisms in the nasal passages that control blood vessel constriction and dilatation. Research in recent years has clarified somewhat the mechanism of mucociliary clearance. Propelled by microscopic, hairlike protrusions called cilia, mucus continually cleanses the nasal membranes. Scientists know that many physiologic factors are involved. Methods of measuring changes in nasal airway resistance are being perfected, which means that the way in which foreign antigens affect the nasal passages should soon be better understood.

Improved understanding of the allergens responsible for rhinitis is a research priority for the future, and the specific reactive parts of many antigens need to be defined. House dust, for example, is a mixture of poorly characterized components. The molecular identification of spores, pollen, and animal dander has just begun. Identification techniques must become more chemical-oriented. Which treatment methods cause the number of antigens to decrease? What is the optimal level of environment control? What are the most efficient and effective methods for removing danders, molds, and pollen from the environment? Someday allergy researchers will have to address themselves to these and similar questions.

The treatment of allergic rhinitis pharmacologically is in the early stages as well. Medications that compete with the mediator histamine at the histamine receptor sites of the nasal mucosa are known as antihistamines. Decongestants are used systematically and topically to shrink blood vessels and thereby decrease fluid leakage and the swelling of membranes. Although effective only for brief periods, topical agents, if overused, can aggravate the nasal membrane swelling already underway. Each of the six families of antihistamine has a different, fundamental chemical structure. If a drug from one family is ineffective in a particular patient, a drug from another family may be tried and found effective. The best-known side effects of antihistamines are drowsiness, dryness of the mouth, and blurred vision. Sometimes combinations of systemic decongestants and antihistamines are used with good results. Topical corticosteroid sprays are a potent adjunct for more serious cases of rhinitis. They are commonly used for brief periods, however, since some degree of systemic absorption occurs, and adrenal gland suppression, a consequence of corticosteroids usage, is a potential adverse effect.

The modification of allergic rhinitis by medication is still of uncertain value. Scientists as yet know little of the relationship of dosage to response for either decongestants or antihistamines. Physicians prescribe the drugs at dosage levels that appear to relieve distress without adverse effects, but neither they nor scientists have determined the optimal dosage for a given individual. Finally, the development of tolerance to these drugs and how long topical corticosteroids can be used safely are still a mystery.

Skin Disease

Allergic skin disease is another research challenge. Atopic dermatitis, or eczema, is an itchy rash which typically starts in early childhood. It is usually, but not always, found in people with other allergic manifestations, such as asthma or rhinitis. Sometimes the disease can be treated successfully by removing or avoiding antigens in the environment, but it is frequently chronic.

Although researchers characterize allergic skin disease as an itchy, scaly red eruption, they know little else about its causes. The extent of their knowledge is that many individuals afflicted by it have defects in cellular immunity, for example, abnormal T cell numbers or abnormal white blood cell mobility toward known chemical attractants (chemotaxis), or both.

What interests many scientists are the natural history of atopic dermatitis and whether the imposition of environmental controls early in a patient's life can alter that history. The use of topical corticosteroids (to decrease inflammation), skin softeners, and antihistamines (to decrease itching) are all being studied.

Many individuals, both allergic and nonallergic, suffer from urticaria, commonly known as hives. Urticaria is an itchy skin eruption characterized by wheals, or small welts, on a flared, red base. Angioedema is a disease characterized by, among other things, swelling of the deep skin layers. Researchers now know that hives occur when mast cells in the skin release the mediator histamine. Histamine causes dilatation of blood vessels, leakage of fluid into the skin layers, and itching. The result is engorgement, wheal formation, redness, and itching.

Research has confirmed that many different stimuli may contribute to the production of hives. Such immunological reactions as those that provoke allergic asthma and rhinitis can become concentrated in the skin, appearing as urticaria; but nonimmunological factors can also trigger the release of histamine by mast cells. Cold; heat; sunlight; systemic disease (for example, rheumatic disease and thyroid disease); certain viral infections; inherited conditions; and possibly psychological factors—all are physical conditions or factors that can provoke hives at certain times in susceptible individuals.

Although histamine has been determined to be the main mediator responsible for hives, other, so-far-undefined mediators probably remain to be discovered. Researchers do not, for example, know how such a variety of nonimmunologic events as physical stimuli, infection, and psychology affect mast cells. What, besides nonimmune events, happens to make mast cells produce histamine, and why are some people and not others stimulated by specific stimuli to develop hives?

Drug Allergy

Drug allergy is a major cause of illness; it sometimes even results in death. Scientific knowledge of the physical characteristics of drugs known to cause allergic reactions is growing, however. The types of drugs most likely to cause reactions are the large, complex molecules, the small molecules that easily link with carrier proteins after administration of a drug, and drugs metabolized to molecules, which also link easily to carrier proteins. Reactions are also classified by type of immunologic reaction: anaphylactic, cytotoxic (cell killing), serum sickness, and cell-mediated immune. In addition, there are nonspecific drug reactions, which, so far, are poorly understood. Because of such factors as genetics, infections, the route of administration, and tissue injury, some people being treated with drugs are at greater risk than others.

It is hoped that research in several areas of drug allergy will soon diminish the number of drug reactions. For example, it may be possible to screen for susceptible reactors by administering predictive tests before a drug is prescribed. For many types of drug, skin and laboratory tests designed to define the drugs that cause particular reactions must be expanded. To accomplish this, research must determine the components and metabolic products that stimulate adverse reactions. Someday, blocking compounds may be available that can thwart an allergic reaction in an individual known to be sensitive to a particular drug.

Stinging Insect Allergy

The Hymenoptera group of insects consists of yellow jackets, bees, wasps, and hornets. Stings from these insects produce dramatic, sometimes life-threatening, reactions in some people. To prevent these reactions, susceptible patients have for years been instructed to carry Adrenalin or antihistamines for immediate use when they are stung. Susceptible people have for some time also taken allergy immunotherapy injections of whole-body extract to obtain protection from future stings.

In recent years, research has demonstrated that venom itself, rather than whole-body extract, is most beneficial for immunotherapy; and venom skin tests can now be given to high-risk individuals. Those identified as being at high risk can be treated using venom injection therapy, which appears to confer blocking antibody and probably changes mast-cell sensitivity, so that people are less likely to have an adverse reaction if stung again.

Although research has led to improved therapy for stinging insect allergy, important questions remain to be answered. Are some people truly protected after the first sting, so that subsequent stings will be harmless even though the initial sting had serious consequences? What is the optimum period for immunotherapy? Can physicians assess a person's clinical response in any way besides another sting?

Immunotherapy

In immunotherapy, also known as hyposensitization or desensitization, a person is injected with antigens to which he or she is allergic, in hopes that he or she will be protected from adverse reactions in the future. Initially, injections are given at frequent intervals, but eventually they are given at longer intervals. The amount of antigen injected increases as treatment progresses. Clinical studies have verified the effectiveness of immunotherapy in reducing the symptoms of allergic rhinitis. In addition, recent evidence suggests that bronchial irritability present in asthma is reduced by immunotherapy. As we saw above, venom immunotherapy appears to diminish the risk of serious reactions to stinging insects.

The mechanism by which immunotherapy relieves symptoms is not yet well understood. Allergy shots appear to stimulate the production of blocking antibodies and to decrease production of allergic antibody. They also appear to change mast-cell sensitivity, so that histamine and other mediators of allergic reactions cannot be released as easily.

Much remains to be learned. The interaction of T and B cells seems to be altered by immunotherapy, thus making it possible for suppressor cells to prevent the production of certain immunoglobulins. This interaction also stimulates helper cells to produce blocking antibodies. Whether this actually occurs remains to be learned. The antigens used in injection therapy need to be standardized, and studies must be made of their effectiveness. Does immunotherapy for rhinitis indeed affect the progression from allergic rhinitis to asthma? Investigators are currently working on "allergoids" for immunotherapy, molecules that, it is hoped, will resemble environmental allergens closely enough to stimulate symptomatic improvement, but without the risk of an allergic reaction. Scientists are also studying compounds that have a sustained action and that have a symptomatic benefit with fewer injections. The goal is to create compounds that require infrequent administration, yet which confer a significant, long-lasting benefit.

Special Problems of Allergic Children

Allergic disease usually appears during childhood. Although it is clear that inherited genetic factors largely determine who will be allergic, little is known about the modulating influence of the genetic code. Current research suggests that viral infections may act as triggers, contributing to a predisposition to allergy in an individual. Perhaps exposure to antigens passed across the placenta, or ingested during the first month of life, influence the course an allergy takes. Researchers have uncovered evidence that suggests that avoidance of certain foods during the early months of life can decrease the incidence of respiratory allergy years later.

In addition to the allergic diseases already mentioned, allergic children seem to experience a specific complication of allergic rhinitis known as Eustachian tube dysfunction. This complication occurs because swollen allergic membranes in the nose and throat impede the normal functioning of the Eustachian tubes, which equalize pressure between the middle ear and the outside world. When the tubes do not function properly, fluid can build up in the middle ears, resulting in recurrent ear infection or hearing loss, or both. If medication and control of environmental allergens do not improve the situation sufficiently, artificial ventilating tubes made of polyethylene must be placed surgically in the tympanic membrane to equalize the pressure. Research in middle ear disease among allergic children is aimed at identifying the scope of the problem, as well as evaluating the various treatments using antihistamines, decongestants, and topical corticosteroids either individually or in combination.

Controversial Research Areas

The Effect of Diet on Behavior

One research area that has stimulated great interest among parents in recent years is the effect of food consumed by children on their behavior. Dr. Ben Feingold, for example, maintains that significant amounts of food dyes and preservatives in a child's diet can contribute to hyperactivity and other types of negative behavior. This claim met with great criticism from the medical community, members of which replied that Dr. Feingold's statements about behavior were sweeping, suggesting that a large proportion of children were being adversely affected; that his observations were not supported by controlled trials, but rather seemed to suggest biased reporting; that the diets recommended by Dr. Feingold were restrictive and difficult to follow, raising the possibility that sacrifices in daily life would be greater than the rewards; and that the term *allergy* had been adopted by followers of the Feingold diet who claimed that children were "allergic" to the dyes and additives, when, in fact, no specific allergens had been noted.

While Dr. Feingold's claims continue to require clarification, and while the criticism remains valid, some investigators have documented that additives and preservatives do increase aberrant behavior in a small group of children considered hyperactive. The mechanism by which these additives work is not an immune or an allergic mechanism, but a toxic one: large doses of the chemicals in additives and preservatives seem to modify nerve function, and certain dyes have been shown to change the releasing of neurotransmitters from the nerves.

Some investigators have reported that the Feingold diet has been effective in a small group of hyperactive children. At the same time, however, research has rejected allergy as the mechanism by which dyes, preservatives, and other chemicals modify behavior. A word of caution is in order. Parents attempting to impose a restrictive diet on their children (or themselves) should be aware of the nutritional deficiencies that can result from the proposed regimen and of the nutritional supplements that should be taken to correct the deficiencies. In a diet that goes beyond simply eliminating "junk food," Dr. Feingold advocates omitting dyes and preservatives; certain fruits, vegetables, and spices; and extracts containing salicylates.

Urine Immunotherapy

Urine immunotherapy is another controversial area of allergy research. Clinics that use it as a treatment have sprung up around the United States. In the therapy, patients bring their own urine to the clinic, where it is filtered and injected back into them. This procedure is purportedly beneficial, but to trained allergists, it is a sham, for which gullible people pay large sums of money despite the lack of evidence supporting the therapy. Belief in such treatment indicates that people have chosen a form of medical treatment without regard for research—the scientific procedures by which medical practices are substantiated and theories verified.

Testing for Food Allergies

Certain methods of testing for and treating food allergies have failed to receive adequate scientific scrutiny. One example is the leukocytotoxic test, which involves putting antigen and serum from an allergic person on a slide with white blood cells. Killed white cells are thought to indicate allergy, but this has not been proved. Other inadequately documented methods are subcutaneous provocation testing and sublingual (under the tongue) provocation testing. In both tests, small amounts of antigen are administered and such side effects as respiratory problems, gastrointestinal problems, irritability, and drowsiness are noted. Because these responses are difficult to relate immunologically to the initial challenge, their validity is questionable.

End-point intracutaneous test titration is an immunotherapy method for determining proper dosage on the basis of the lowest concentration of antigen that produces a specific wheal. Essentially, the technique is low-dose immunotherapy. It differs from conventional immunotherapy only in that, instead of giving as large an antigen load as is feasible to produce immunologic protection, the smallest feasible dose is given. This method was recently compared with conventional immunotherapy for ragweed hay fever, and was found less effective.

Psychosomatic Aspects of Allergy

Anyone prone to allergy spends a lot of time asking—and trying to answer—such questions as, Are allergies all in my head? Does my child deliberately make himself wheeze? Why does my nose always get stuffy when I'm nervous?

Allergic diseases are not figments of the imagination. Once a person becomes disposed to allergic disease, however, many factors may be involved in aggravating the individual's physical problem. People with asthma have overly sensitive and reactive muscles in the bronchial tree, just as patients with allergic rhinitis have overly sensitive blood vessels and mucous-secreting cells in the nose. When these individuals are faced with such stresses as exposure to allergens, irritating fumes, or viral infections, their allergic problems may well increase. This is not a deliberate turning on of reactivity, but rather a manifestation of increased reactivity to various stimuli by the allergic end-organ. Just as a man with an ulcer can aggravate his difficulties by eating spicy foods or allowing the pressure of work to upset him, an asthmatic who breathes in pollen or who has a stressful work situation can suffer bronchospasm. The physical raw material responsible for the ulcer or the asthma, however, existed before the stressful situation and determined the course the stress would take.

The extent to which an allergic individual can control reactions to external factors has a lot to do with the individual's coping mechanism—how secure the person is, whether he enjoys his job, how much pleasure he derives from daily chores, and so on. It is important that the physician explain this interaction of physical disease and environment (both psychological and physical) to the allergic person. That way, the link between what the person thinks and feels, and his or her physical problems, is less likely to be misconstrued as a psychosomatic, attention-getting mechanism.

The allergy sufferer should not lose sight of the tremendous psychological impact a person with a significant allergy problem has on the people around him. Someone with severe eczema may be viewed as ugly and unfortunate, as someone to be avoided. People may misunderstand the medical problem and consider it infectious and dangerous to their health if they associate too closely with the allergy sufferer. A person with asthma may be considered an invalid who cannot participate in normal activities. The person's family or spouse may be annoyed, or even angry, because of coughing fits that disturb sleep, physical limitations that force daily lives to be altered, medical costs that prohibit other spending.

Allergic individuals undoubtedly can encourage negative feelings in people around them if these people remain ignorant of allergy problems. With education comes understanding that can help the allergic patient, as well as the patient's friends and family, cope with allergy problems. Knowledge of allergies helps them understand that allergic disease is not a will-o'-the-wisp but a physical ailment that can be affected either positively or negatively by the environment. For example, exposure to cigarette smoke, paint fumes, or freshly mowed grass can exacerbate an individual's control, and avoidance of compounds known to be noxious or threatening can subdue allergic reactivity.

There are several ways of correcting negative ways of coping with difficulties (for example, a bad experience always provokes wheezing). One is to observe the cause-and-effect relationship between an event and a negative result. Sometimes a friend or a physician merely has to suggest such a relationship to someone for them to understand their behavior and correct it. In the case of a complex allergy problem, the allergy victim may not admit a problem or may not be able to correct an annoying reaction pattern. Counselling by a professional psychiatrist, a psychologist, or a primary-care physician can sometimes correct the behavioral pattern. Behavioral modification and biofeedback methods can also alter reaction patterns in some situations.

Summary

Whether it is in the field of epidemiology, the research laboratory, or the clinical laboratory, progress is being made in increasing the fund of scientific knowledge about allergy problems and what to do about them. The various facets of research are of more or less equal importance. Population studies are done to increase awareness of the dimensions of allergy problems. While investigators in the laboratory study the molecular basis of the mechanisms that cause problems, clinicians observe and suggest possible pharmacological adjustments to correct them. Both animals and humans are tested. There is, indeed, a research chain; each link must be strong if knowledge is to be expanded.

Ultimately, research must be translated into practical results. Scientists, physicians, patients, and their families must be able to use the products of research. One of the ways to make sure that this happens is through education and dissemination of information about research, treatment, and new products. For that purpose, The Asthma & Allergy Foundation of America offers reference materials, trained physicians to answer questions, and literature such as this book. Community lung associations offer courses designed to increase understanding of allergic diseases. Summer camps and residential services exist for allergic children; they are designed to teach the children about their problems and help them lead more normal lives. Thanks to research and its application in everyday life, allergic disease, albeit often chronic, can be better understood, modified, and controlled.

References

Frick, O. L. "Controversial Concepts and Techniques, with Emphasis on Food Allergy." In *Allergic Diseases of Infancy, Childhood and Adolescence,* ed. C. W. Bierman and D. S. Pearlman. Philadelphia: W. B. Saunders, 1980.

Furukawa, C. T., and Roesler, T. A. "Psychological Aspects of Allergic Disease." In *Allergic Diseases of Infancy, Childhood and Adolescence,* ed. C. W. Bierman and D. S. Pearlman. Philadelphia: W. B. Saunders, 1980.

General Considerations for Clinical Evaluation of Drugs. FDA publication 77-3040.

NIAID Task Force Report. *Asthma and the Other Allergic Diseases.* NIH Publication No. 79, 387, May 1979.

Van Metre, T. E., et al. "A Controlled Study of the Effectiveness of the Rinkel Method of Immunotherapy for Ragweed Pollen Hay Fever." *Journal of Allergy and Clinical Immunology,* 65:288, 1980.

CHAPTER 7

Regional Factors in Allergy
by William R. Solomon, M.D.

When allergic people travel or move to other regions of the country, their symptoms may change, and most often these variations are caused by regional differences in pollen-producing plants. Other factors, however, including airborne fungus spores, algae, and insect fragments, as well as food components, also can vary from place to place and affect a patient's health accordingly. At times, desired symptom improvements do not occur despite carefully planned major geographic moves. In effect, allergens from domestic dust, bedding, upholstery, and house pets accompany the patient and continue to provoke illness in the new surroundings. These factors, reflecting household practices and life style, have indoor or job-related sources and can be effectively eliminated by applying practical environmental measures.

Allergic symptoms also may recur in distant places because of acquired sensitivity to allergens (for example, pollens) unique to the new area. More often, the disappointed patient has simply not yet left the range of an offender allergen despite a journey of hundreds or even sometimes thousands of miles. As many grasses and tree species, for example, grow throughout the continent, avoidance of their pollens is difficult and requires careful selection of refuge areas. Thus, permanent geographic moves to change allergen exposure should not be undertaken impulsively. They might be considered after successful trial periods in the area under consideration.

While allergic problems may be difficult to predict in a new area, some estimate of expected allergen exposure is possible. The following charts should assist such speculation as well as indicate the allergens that may produce recurrent symptoms in established regional populations.

To simplify reference, groups of states and bordering Canadian provinces with similar climate and pollen allergens are considered together. As the resulting groupings are large and not strictly uniform,

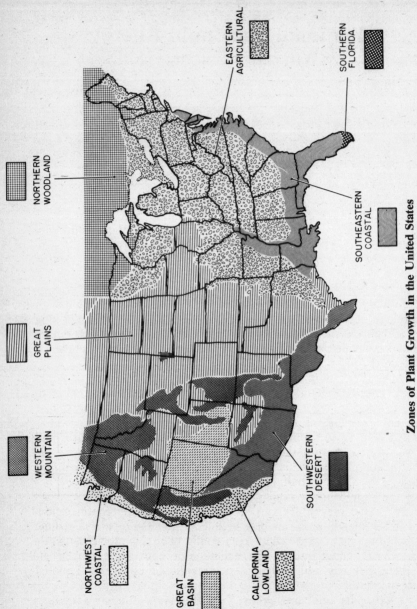

Zones of Plant Growth in the United States
(See charts in accompanying chapter for explanation of zones.)

these charts only describe average conditions. Points close to a boundary between two areas will, of course, have allergens typical of both.

For each region, important hay fever plants are listed with the time of pollen shedding for each indicated with respect to the calendar year, with the horizontal bars across the columns indicating the time of the allergen occurrence. Plants that are mostly cultivated are marked (C), and sources restricted to part of a region are denoted by (N) North, (S) South, (E) East, (W) West, (L) Local, and (NW) Northwest.

In each table, noteworthy pollen-producing trees are noted first, followed by grasses, and broad-leafed plants without woody stems (or weeds). For each type, an approximate indication of the importance of an allergy offender in the overall region is given on a scale ranging from ± (minor) to +++ (very major).

The reader should understand that these appraisals are overall averages for entire regions and their allergic populations. Differences in individual sensitivities and the local distribution of sources (such as pollen-producing plants) may convert a generally unimportant pollen type into a major cause of symptoms.

NORTHERN WOODLAND	JAN.	FEB.	MARCH	APRIL	MAY	JUNE	JULY	AUG.	SEPT.	OCT.	NOV.	DEC.	
Hazelnut				▓	▓								±
Aspen, Poplar				▓	▓								+
Alder				▓	▓								+
Birch				▓	▓								++
Willow				▓	▓								+
Grasses, Sedges						▓	▓						±

Other factors—Pine, spruce, fir, and hemlock pollens are released in large amounts but are not proven factors in hay fever and asthma. Some ragweed occurs where the forest has been disturbed. Fungi—especially mushrooms and puffballs—are abundant (June–October) but seem to cause only limited symptoms. Cabins and cottages that have been left closed for many months and that are often not fully watertight tend to be moldy.

Tables on pages 140–153 adapted from material originally appearing in *A Manual of Clinical Allergy*, J. M. Sheldon, R. G. Lovell, and K. P. Mathews, editors and reprinted by permission of W. B. Saunders, Philadelphia, PA. Copyright © 1953.

EASTERN AGRICULTURAL

	JAN.	FEB.	MARCH	APRIL	MAY	JUNE	JULY	AUG.	SEPT.	OCT.	NOV.	DEC.		
Red Cedar		■	■											+
Hazelnut			■											±
Elm			■											+++
Alder			■											+
Aspen, Poplar			■											+
Box Elder			■	■									W	+++
Maple*				■	■									±
Birch				■										++
Bayberry, Wax Myrtle				■	■	■							L	+
Ash				■										++
Sweet Gum				■									SE	+
Paper Mulberry				■									S	+
Willow			■	■	■									±
Sycamore				■										++
Beech				■	■									+
Oak					■									++
Hackberry					■								L	+
Mulberry (Red)					■									++
Hickory					■									+
Walnut					■									++
Grasses					■	■	■							+++
Red (Sheep) Sorrel					■	■								+
Plantain					■	■								±
Nettle						■								+
Hemp							■	■					NW	++
Ragweed, Marsh Elder							■	■						+++
Sage							■	■					W	+
Goosefoot, Amaranth							■	■	■					++

*Types besides box elder

Other factors—Insect scales and hairs may provoke symptoms in such localities as inland lakes where certain types swarm seasonally. Fungi are important factors from May to November, especially in grain-growing areas; exposure increases whenever vegetation or soil is disturbed. Plants that process seed materials—such as castor bean, cottonseed, and soybean—may release dusts that cause allergic reactions.

SOUTHEASTERN COASTAL

	JAN.	FEB.	MARCH	APRIL	MAY	JUNE	JULY	AUG.	SEPT.	OCT.	NOV.	DEC.		
Red Cedar		▓	▓											+
Hackberry		▓	▓	▓									L	+
Elm		▓	▓											++
Willow			▓	▓										±
Poplar			▓	▓										+
Bald Cypress			▓	▓										±
Bayberry, Wax Myrtle			▓	▓									L	±
Ash			▓	▓										++
Birch			▓											+
Pecan (C), Hickory		▓	▓	▓										++
Paper Mulberry (C)			▓	▓										+
Sycamore				▓										++
Mulberry			▓	▓										+
Oak			▓	▓										+++
Walnut				▓										+
Grasses		▓	▓	▓	▓	▓	▓	▓	▓	▓				+++
Red (Sheep) Sorrel, Dock					▓	▓								+
Plantain					▓	▓	▓	▓						±
Nettle					▓	▓	▓							±
Sage						▓	▓	▓					L	±
Ragweed, Marsh Elder								▓	▓					+++
Goosefoot, Amaranth						▓	▓	▓						+

Other factors—Fungus exposures can produce symptoms during much of the year. High humidity encourages fungus growth and may directly affect respiratory symptoms.

SOUTHERN FLORIDA

	JAN.	FEB.	MARCH	APRIL	MAY	JUNE	JULY	AUG.	SEPT.	OCT.	NOV.	DEC.	
Oak		▓	▓	▓									++
Bald Cypress	▓	▓	▓	▓									±
Maple	▓	▓	▓	▓									±
Elm			▓	▓									+
Bayberry, Wax Myrtle			▓								L		±
Australian Pine			▓										+
Pecan, Hickory			▓	▓									+
Mulberry			▓	▓									+
Grasses	▓	▓	▓	▓	▓	▓	▓	▓	▓	▓	▓		++
Ragweed, Marsh Elder						▓	▓	▓	▓	▓	▓		++
Sorrel, Dock					▓	▓	▓	▓	▓	▓	▓		±
Goosefoot, Amaranth					▓	▓	▓	▓	▓	▓	▓		±

Other factors—Pollens from eucalyptus, Brazilian pepper tree, palms, and other cultivated trees occur but are probably minor factors at most. Fungus spores in moderate numbers are airborne throughout the year, and indoor fungus growth is fostered by the continuously high relative humidity.

GREAT PLAINS

	JAN.	FEB.	MARCH	APRIL	MAY	JUNE	JULY	AUG.	SEPT.	OCT.	NOV.	DEC.		
Mountain Cedar, Juniper	■	■	■										W	+
Elm		■	■	■										+
Ash			■	■										+
Oak		■	■	■										++
Poplar		■	■	■										+
Box Elder			■	■										+
Willow			■	■										±
Hackberry				■									S	+
Sycamore			■	■										+
Hickory, Pecan				■	■									+
Mulberry				■										+
Osage Orange				■									SE	±
Grasses				■	■	■	■	■	■					++
Sorrel, Dock					■	■	■							±
Hemp							■	■						+
Goosefoot, Amaranth						■	■	■	■					+++
Ragweed, Marsh Elder								■	■					+++
Sage								■	■	■			W	++

Other factors—Extensive livestock operations provide local sources of animal dander exposure. In addition, dusts from fertilizers and animal feeds, as well as from grain-storage facilities, can create serious allergic problems. Cultivated areas are especially important sources of fungus spores from early summer to the first snowfall.

WESTERN MOUNTAIN

	JAN.	FEB.	MARCH	APRIL	MAY	JUNE	JULY	AUG.	SEPT.	OCT.	NOV.	DEC.		
Mountain Cedar, Juniper													SE	+++
Elm														+
Alder														±
Maple														+
Ash														±
Willow														±
Aspen, Poplar														+
Birch														+
Oak													S	+
Walnut														+
Grasses														++
Ragweed													E	+++
Sage													L	++
Goosefoot, Amaranth														+++

Other factors—In this region, huge amounts of pollen are released by conifers—including pines, spruce, fir, and hemlocks—but their effect on allergic people remains in dispute. Fungus spores derived from field crops are less abundant than in areas located farther east.

GREAT BASIN

	JAN.	FEB.	MARCH	APRIL	MAY	JUNE	JULY	AUG.	SEPT.	OCT.	NOV.	DEC.	
Juniper		▓	▓	▓									+
Elm			▓	▓									±
Poplar			▓	▓									+
Willow			▓	▓									±
Sycamore				▓	▓								±
Box Elder				▓									±
Grasses					▓	▓	▓	▓					+
Sage						▓	▓	▓	▓				++
Goosefoot, Amaranth							▓	▓	▓				++
Ragweed							▓	▓	▓				+

Other factors—In hilly areas, birch, aspen, and oak pollens may cause seasonal allergy. Fungus exposures are only rarely a source of major symptoms.

SOUTHWESTERN DESERT	JAN.	FEB.	MARCH	APRIL	MAY	JUNE	JULY	AUG.	SEPT.	OCT.	NOV.	DEC.		
Mountain Cedar	▨	▨	▨									▨	E	+++
Arizona Cypress		▨	▨											++
Elm		▨	▨											+
Ash		▨	▨											+
Poplar		▨	▨											+
Mulberry			▨	▨										++
Olive			▨	▨	▨									+
Grasses			▨	▨	▨	▨	▨	▨	▨	▨				++
Sugar Beet (C)								▨	▨				L	±
Ragweed				▨	▨			▨	▨	▨				++
Goosefoot, Amaranth			▨	▨				▨	▨	▨				++
Sage			▨	▨				▨	▨	▨				+

Other factors—Pollen produced by tamarisks and mesquite or by plantings of castor bean, pecan, or eucalyptus may, in rare instances, produce respiratory allergy. Fungus exposures are relatively low, although extensive irrigation promotes fungus growth. The use of evaporative ("swamp") cooling units in buildings increases indoor fungus exposure, although the risks involved are not precisely known.

154 □ THE ALLERGY ENCYCLOPEDIA

CALIFORNIA LOWLAND

	JAN.	FEB.	MARCH	APRIL	MAY	JUNE	JULY	AUG.	SEPT.	OCT.	NOV.	DEC.		
Mulberry		■	■	■										+
Alder		■	■											±
Ash		■	■	■										+
Willow		■	■	■	■									±
Walnut (C)			■	■									L	±
Cottonwood (Poplar)			■	■										+
Elm		■	■											+
Sycamore			■	■										+
Oak			■	■										+
Birch			■	■										±
Olive (C)				■	■								S	±
Grasses			■	■	■	■	■	■	■	■	■			++
Ragweed							■	■	■					±
Sage							■	■	■	■				+
Goosefoot, Amaranth							■	■	■					+

Other factors—The effects produced by eucalyptus, coast maple, and acacia pollens are unknown. Fungus exposures vary from mild to moderate according to the density of local plant cover.

NORTHWEST COASTAL	JAN.	FEB.	MARCH	APRIL	MAY	JUNE	JULY	AUG.	SEPT.	OCT.	NOV.	DEC.		
Incense Cedar	■	■											L	+
Hazelnut (C)	■	■												+
Alder		■	■	■										±
Willow		■	■	■										±
Ash			■	■										+
Box Elder			■	■										±
Birch				■										+
Aspen, Poplar				■										+
Elm			■	■										+
Maple				■										±
Oak				■										+
Walnut				■	■									+
Grasses					■	■	■	■	■					++
Plantain					■	■	■	■						+
Red Sorrel					■	■								±
Goosefoot, Amaranth					■	■	■	■	■					++
Ragweed							■	■	■				L	±

Other factors—Areas devoted to grass-seed production may experience high grass-pollen levels as a result. Large amounts of conifer pollen are shed, especially at higher elevations, but they are generally of uncertain importance in allergy. Respiratory illnesses, including asthma, are associated with wood industries, most notably where western red cedar is processed. Fungi flourish in humid coastal areas; the types present, however, seem to cause milder symptoms than does exposure in grain-growing areas of eastern regions.

Additional Areas

Alaska

Respiratory allergy is, at most, a minor problem for persons living in arctic and subarctic areas. In most areas, brief periods of pollen-shedding by birches, alders, and willows precede a short grass-pollen "season." Although the levels of fungus spores seem to be comparatively low, animal dander, especially dog dander, often is a prominent exposure factor throughout the year.

Hawaii

Airborne grass pollen probably is the most widespread causative agent in allergy, with exposure occurring during much of the year. As is true of most tropical and subtropical areas, few trees shed significant amounts of wind-borne pollen; acacia, eucalyptus, or "Australian pine" (*Casuarina*) pollen is, however, occasionally suspected of causing an allergy. Fungus exposure is prominent both indoors and out of doors and is responsible for symptoms in many allergic persons.

Puerto Rico

Clearly, grasses are the major source of pollen allergy, regardless of the time of year. Also, significant levels of fungus spores, accompanied by allergic symptoms, occur in all the seasons. It is suspected, too, that insect-derived material plays a role in allergies. One source of insect debris is the droppings of bats, which often live in the roofs of private homes. It is not clear, though, whether the droppings contain bat dander. Respiratory irritation from the smoke of burning sugar cane is widely recognized, but a true allergy to the smoke has not been proved.

POLLEN CALENDAR

Months: JAN. / FEB. / MARCH / APRIL / MAY / JUNE / JULY / AUG. / SEPT. / OCT. / NOV. / DEC.

ALABAMA — Montgomery
- TREE: Jan.–April
- GRASS: May–Sept.
- RAG.: Sept.–Oct.

ARIZONA — Phoenix
- TREE: Feb.–April
- RAG.: Sept.–Oct.
- GRASS: May–Oct.
- RAG.: March–May
- AMARANTH: June–Oct.

Kingman
- R. T.-SALT BUSH: June–Sept.
- RAGWEED: Aug.–Sept.

ARKANSAS — Little Rock
- TREE: Feb.–April
- GRASS: May–Sept.
- RAG.: Sept.–Oct.

CALIFORNIA — Northwestern
- TREE: March–June
- RAGWEED-SAGE: July–Oct.
- GRASS: April–Sept.
- CHENOPOD-SALT BUSH: April–Sept.

Southern
- TREE: Feb.–March
- RUSSIAN THISTLE: July–Oct.
- GRASS: April–Oct.
- RAGWEED-SAGE: July–Oct.

San Francisco Bay
- TREE: Feb.–May
- RAGWEED-SAGE: June–Sept.
- GRASS: April–Nov.
- DOCK-PLANTAIN: May–June

COLORADO — Denver
- TREE: April–May
- SAGE: Aug.–Sept.
- R. THIS.-KOCHIA: June–Sept.
- GRASS: May–June
- RAG.: Aug.–Sept.

CONNECTICUT
- TREE: March–May
- GRASS: May–June
- RAG.: Sept.–Oct.

DELAWARE
- TREE: March–May
- GRASS: May–June
- RAG.: Aug.–Oct.

DIST. OF COL. — Washington
- TREE: March–May
- GRASS: May–June
- RAG.: Aug.–Oct.

FLORIDA — Miami
- TREE: Jan.–March
- GRASS: March–June
- RAGWEED: June–Aug.
- GRASS: Aug.–Dec.

Tampa
- TREE: Feb.–April
- GRASS: Jan.–Dec.
- RAG.: Sept.–Oct.

GEORGIA — Atlanta
- TREE: Feb.–April
- GRASS: May–Aug.
- RAG.: Sept.–Oct.

POLLEN CALENDAR (Continued)

Months: JAN. | FEB. | MARCH | APRIL | MAY | JUNE | JULY | AUG. | SEPT. | OCT. | NOV. | DEC.

IDAHO — Southern
- TREE: March–May
- SAGE: Aug.–Sept.
- R.T.-SALT BUSH: July–Sept.
- GRASS: May–June
- RAG.: Sept.

ILLINOIS — Chicago
- TREE: April–May
- GRASS: May–June
- RAG.: Aug.–Sept.

INDIANA — Indianapolis
- TREE: April–May
- GRASS: May–June
- RAG.: Aug.–Sept.

IOWA — Ames
- TREE: April–May
- GRASS: June–Aug.
- RAG.: Sept.

KANSAS — Wichita
- TREE: March–May
- GRASS: May–June
- R.T.-AMAR.: Aug.–Sept.
- RAG.: Sept.–Oct.

KENTUCKY — Louisville
- TREE: March–May
- GRASS: June–July
- RAG.: Sept.

LOUISIANA — New Orleans
- TREE: Feb.–March
- GRASS: April–Oct.
- RAGWEED: Aug.–Oct.

MAINE
- TREE: April–May
- GRASS: May–June
- RAG.: Aug.–Sept.

MARYLAND — Baltimore
- TREE: March–April
- GRASS: May–June
- RAG.: Aug.–Sept.

MASS. — Boston
- TREE: April–May
- GRASS: May–June
- RAG.: Aug.–Sept.

MICHIGAN — Detroit
- TREE: April–May
- GRASS: May–June
- RAG.: Aug.–Sept.

MINNESOTA — Minneapolis
- TREE: April–May
- CHEN.-AMAR.: June–July
- GRASS: June–July
- RAG.: Aug.–Sept.

MISSISSIPPI — Vicksburg
- TREE: March–April
- GRASS: May–Aug.
- RAG.: Sept.

MISSOURI — St. Louis / Kansas City
- TREE: April–May
- CH.-AMAR.: July–Aug.
- GRASS: May–June
- RAG.: Sept.

POLLEN CALENDAR (Continued)

Location / Pollen	JAN.	FEB.	MARCH	APRIL	MAY	JUNE	JULY	AUG.	SEPT.	OCT.	NOV.	DEC.
MONTANA — Miles City												
TREE				■	■							
RAG.-SAGE								■	■			
GRASS					■	■	■	■				
R. THISTLE							■	■				
NEBRASKA — Omaha												
TREE			■	■	■							
R. THISTLE							■	■				
GRASS						■	■					
HEMP							■	■				
RAG.								■	■			
NEVADA — Reno												
TREE				■	■							
RAG.								■	■			
GRASS					■	■	■					
SAGE								■	■			
R. T.-SALT BUSH						■	■	■	■			
NEW HAMPSHIRE												
TREE				■	■							
GRASS					■	■	■					
RAG.								■	■			
NEW JERSEY												
TREE				■	■							
GRASS					■	■	■					
RAG.								■	■			
NEW MEXICO — Roswell												
TREE			■	■	■	■	■	■				
R.-SAGE									■	■		
GRASS					■	■	■	■	■			
AMAR.-SALT BUSH						■	■	■				
NEW YORK — New York City												
TREE				■	■							
GRASS					■	■	■					
RAG.								■	■			
NO. CAROLINA — Raleigh												
TREE		■	■	■								
GRASS					■	■	■					
RAG.								■	■			
NORTH DAKOTA — Fargo												
TREE				■	■							
R. THISTLE							■	■				
GRASS						■	■					
SAGE								■	■			
RAGWEED							■	■				
OHIO — Cleveland												
TREE				■	■							
GRASS						■	■					
RAG.								■	■			
OKLAHOMA — Oklahoma City												
TREE			■	■	■							
AMARANTH						■	■	■				
GRASS					■	■	■	■				
RAG.								■	■			
OREGON — Portland												
TREE				■	■							
GRASS						■	■	■				
DOCK-PLANTAIN						■	■	■	■			
OREGON — East of Cascade Mountains												
TREE				■	■							
GRASS						■	■					
SAGE								■	■			
R.T.-SALT BUSH							■	■	■			
RAG.								■	■			
PENNSYLVANIA												
TREE				■	■							
GRASS					■	■	■					
RAG.								■	■			

POLLEN CALENDAR (Continued)

	JAN.	FEB.	MARCH	APRIL	MAY	JUNE	JULY	AUG.	SEPT.	OCT.	NOV.	DEC.
RHODE ISLAND				TREE	TREE							
					GRASS	GRASS	GRASS					
								RAG.	RAG.			
SO. CAROLINA Charleston			TREE	TREE								
					GRASS	GRASS	GRASS					
								RAGWEED	RAGWEED	RAGWEED		
SOUTH DAKOTA				TREE	TREE							
						GRASS	GRASS					
							R. THISTLE	R. THISTLE				
								SAGE	SAGE			
								RAGWEED	RAGWEED			
TENNESSEE Nashville			TREE	TREE	TREE							
						GRASS	GRASS	GRASS				
									SAGE			
									ELM			
								ELM				
TEXAS Dallas		TREE	TREE	TREE								
								ELM	ELM			
					GRASS	GRASS	GRASS	GRASS				
									RAGWEED	RAGWEED		
Brownsville	GRASS	GRASS	GRASS	GRASS	GRASS	GRASS	GRASS	GRASS	GRASS	GRASS		
				HACKBERRY	HACKBERRY							
								AMARANTH	AMARANTH			
						RAGWEED	RAGWEED	RAGWEED	RAGWEED	RAGWEED		
UTAH Salt Lake City				TREE	TREE							
							R. THISTLE	R. THISTLE				
					GRASS	GRASS	GRASS					
								SAGE	SAGE			
								RAG.				
VERMONT				TREE	TREE							
					GRASS	GRASS						
								RAG.				
VIRGINIA Richmond			TREE	TREE	TREE							
						GRASS	GRASS					
								RAG.				
WASHINGTON Seattle			TREE	TREE								
						GRASS	GRASS	GRASS	GRASS			
						DOCK-PLANTAIN	DOCK-PLANTAIN	DOCK-PLANTAIN	DOCK-PLANTAIN			
Eastern				TREE	TREE							
									SAGE			
						GRASS	GRASS					
								R.T.-SALT BUSH	R.T.-SALT BUSH			
									RAG.			
WEST VIRGINIA				TREE	TREE							
					GRASS	GRASS						
								RAG.				
WISCONSIN Madison				TREE	TREE							
						GRASS	GRASS					
								RAG.				
WYOMING				TREE	TREE							
						GRASS	GRASS					
								SAGE	SAGE			
							R. THISTLE	R. THISTLE				
							RAGWEED	RAGWEED				

CHAPTER 8

Food Allergies
and Allergy Cooking

If you are an allergy patient or the parent of an allergic child, the information presented in this chapter should help you understand better some of the more common problems involved in food allergy and cooking for those with food allergies. Before following *any* of the advice given in this chapter, however, check with your allergy physician to see whether it is appropriate for your particular situation.

Food Allergies

What exactly is food allergy?

Although food allergy was first studied scientifically only half a century ago, the Egyptians, Chinese, Jews, Greeks, and Romans of antiquity were aware that, as Lucretius observed over 2,100 years ago, "One man's meat is another man's poison." Some biblical scholars believe the Old Testament's dietary restrictions reflected, in many instances, an awareness that certain foods caused severe symptoms in some people.

Food allergy is a specific food hypersensitivity that develops when the offending (allergenic) substance happens to be a food. The symptoms that develop after eating a certain food or foods can involve the skin, the nasal passages, the respiratory or gastrointestinal tract, and very rarely the entire circulatory system.

There are two major types of allergenic reaction to foods: immediate and delayed. The immediate reaction is often violent and sometimes life-threatening. The symptoms appear within minutes after the food has been eaten, and sometimes even before it is swallowed. This is particularly true of patients allergic to shellfish, nuts, and eggs. On the other hand, delayed reactions to foods are subtler, as it may be many hours before the symptoms appear. Thus, it is much more difficult for patients to associate their symptoms with a particular food substance. It is generally believed that in the immediate reaction the offending food is the whole protein while in the delayed reaction some substance formed during the digestive process is involved.

Who is most likely to suffer from food allergy?

Anyone with a tendency to allergy generally can be, or become, sensitive to one or more foods. The tendency to allergy is inherited; it can show up in any symptoms of allergy, and any substance can become the sensitizer, including foods. A child has a 75 percent chance of developing an allergy at an early age if both his parents are allergic.

Although food allergy can occur at just about any age, it is most likely to appear during infancy. As children grow older, their food allergies often change; such children may develop an allergy to a new food, or lose an existing allergy. Most food allergies, however, are outgrown.

What are the most common symptoms of food allergy?

Food allergy symptoms can involve specific organs and systems of the body and sometimes every organ and system. In the respiratory system, food allergy can cause asthma (manifested by coughing and wheezing) and such nasal symptoms as itching, runny nose, sneezing, snorting, and phlegm in the throat. Diarrhea, nausea, or vomiting, and bellyache or cramps (colic in infants) may develop when food allergy affects the digestive system.

Any area of the body may be subjected to swelling (edema), including the eyes, lips, face, and tongue. If the swelling develops in the throat and upper windpipe, breathing can be seriously impaired and suffocation may result. Eczema, a chronic skin disease, can sometimes also be caused by food allergy, and a rash may form in the bends of the arms and possibly all over the body.

Food allergy can also cause fluid to develop behind the eardrums, which may result in intermittent deafness. Other symptoms sometimes caused by food allergy are migraine headaches, a mottled tongue, and canker sores in the mouth. It has been suggested, although not yet proved, that hyperactivity, irritability, and aggressiveness in children may also result from food allergy.

Immediate reactions to food affecting the throat and respiratory passages are particularly dangerous. Patients experiencing shock in response to an allergenic food usually develop severe nausea, vomiting, hives, and swellings all over the body and may collapse. These immediate allergic reactions can be life-threatening; they require instant attention.

Table 8.1 is a list of symptoms sometimes caused by food allergy, though they may also be caused by other factors:

Table 8.1. List of Symptoms

DIGESTIVE UPSET	SKIN
Vomiting	Hives
Nausea	Eczema
Cramps	Canker sores
Indigestion	Inflammation of lips
Belching	Inflammation of
Constipation	inside of mouth
Diarrhea	Itchy skin
Abdominal distention	Itchy anus
Stomach ache	Itchy eyes
Appendicitislike symptoms	Excessive sweating
	Swelling of glands
	(neck especially)
	Pallor

NERVOUS SYSTEM	OTHER
Migraine	Asthma
One-side headache	Rhinitis (runny nose)
Spots before eyes	Dizziness
Listlessness	Earaches
Hyperactivity	Urinary frequency
Lack of concentration	Bed-wetting
Tension-fatigue syndrome	Fatigue
Irritability	Arthritis
Intermittent headaches	Hoarseness
Nervous tension	Muscle aching
Tiredness	Low-grade fever
Chilliness	

How is food allergy diagnosed?

Even if one or more of the symptoms associated with food allergy is present, a food allergy may not be responsible. The same symptoms may be caused by food spoilage or contamination, by the method of cooking or feeding, by the body's lack of an enzyme or some other digestive factor, or simply by digestive intolerance. Other causes are internal diseases involving the stomach, gall bladder, intestines, and pancreas, as well as fatigue, stress, drugs, and emotional problems.

Once these possibilities have been ruled out, the food allergy patient is ready for a rigorous diagnostic process, the first step of which is a careful history. This may be followed by skin testing. Unfortunately, however, although such tests are reliable in diagnosing allergies to dust, pollen, or pets, they are less so in diagnosing the specific cause of a food allergy. Test extracts made from food tend to lose their potency fairly quickly; they often fail to provoke a skin reaction in case of proven sensitivity. Though the tests may be positive in people experiencing immediate reactions to allergenic foods, they are considered, in many cases, to be without clinical significance.

Skin tests are even less reliable among patients experiencing the delayed type of reaction, as the test extract contains only the whole food and no digested material—though the latter is usually involved in this kind of reaction.

Another testing method involves placing diluted food extracts under the tongue, but this method is also considered unreliable and is often omitted. Treatment by administering extract solutions under the tongue is also not a warranted method.

A trial diet is the most effective procedure known for determining the specific food or foods to which a patient is allergic. On the first day, the patient eats the suspected offending food in all forms and in substantial quantities, provoking an allergic response. Then, for the next five days, the suspected offending food is avoided totally, which should result in an absence of symptoms. On day seven, the suspected offending food is again eaten, on an empty stomach, and in its pure form (that is, for example, a glass of milk, but not cheese or ice cream). The pattern of reaction and nonreaction will either be significant enough to eliminate all doubt about the effect of the food or the suspected food will be eliminated from consideration as the cause of the allergic reaction.

What testing methods are used when the patient has no idea what food he or she is allergic to?

Two general procedures are resorted to in this case:

1. Symptoms that occur only once in a while may be caused by infrequently eaten foods. A food allergy patient can sometimes help to determine the offending food by keeping a "food diary" in which each food eaten, the time of day, and any symptoms noted, are set down. Any medicines taken orally and any known exposure to environmental pollutants must also be recorded.

A sample food diary is reproduced below. To determine the offending food, those foods that are believed to produce symptoms are checked individually by eliminating them from the diet for a week and then eating them in substantial amounts.

2. When symptoms occur every day, a special elimination diet, including at first only foods seldom found to cause allergy, may be prescribed. One by one, suspect foods are then added to the diet. When the symptoms occur regularly after a specific food is eaten, that food must be eliminated from the patient's diet.

Figure 8.1.   Sample Food Diary

	First Day	Second Day	Third Day	Fourth Day	Fifth Day	Sixth Day	Seventh Day
BREAKFAST							
Symptoms							
Medication							
LUNCH							
Symptoms							
Medication							
DINNER							
Symptoms							
Medication							

What foods are allergenic (cause allergenic sensitivity)?

Any food can cause an allergenic reaction, but such foods as tree nuts, peanuts, shellfish, chocolate, and strawberries are more often allergenic than others. The excessive ingestion of a food sometimes creates sensitivity to that food. Thus, Scandinavians are most commonly allergic to fish, the Japanese to rice. In the American diet, frequently eaten, and thus frequently allergenic, foods include milk, eggs, wheat, gluten, corn, and soya.

A person allergic to one food is frequently allergic to related foods. For example, peanuts belong to the legume family, and people allergic to them often cannot eat peas and beans. They are not necessarily allergic, however, to all nuts, which fall into eleven different botanical families. By the same token, patients allergic to wheat are often allergic to other grains, but not necessarily to buckwheat, part of a different botanical family. Potatoes are related to tomatoes, but not to sweet potatoes.

The following chart, which also includes many garden and medicinal plants in common usage, indicates the botanical families to which various occasionally allergenic food substances belong.

Table 8.2. Botanical List of Food Families

FAMILY	FOOD	RELATED PLANTS, EXTRACTS OR ALTERNATE IDENTIFICATION
*Apple (Malus)	Apple (cider, pectin), Crabapple	
*Berry (Rubus)	Blackberry, Boysenberry, Dewberry, Loganberry, Raspberry, Saskatoon Berry, Youngberry	Bramble
*Pear (Pyrus)	Pear	
*Plum (Prunus)	Almond, Apricot, Cherry, Nectarine, Peach, Plum, Prune	
*Quince (Haenomeles)	Quince (pectin)	Japanese Quince
Rose	Blackthorn (Sloe), Strawberry, Loquat, Medlar	Rose, Woodruff, Sweetbrier, Cinquefoil, Hawthorn
Amaryllis		Amaryllis, Belladonna Lily, Daffodil
Ammoniacum		Gum Ammoniacum, Spirits of Ammonia
Arum	Poi, Taro, Dasheen	Arum, Jack-in-the-Pulpit
Balsam		Frankincense, Olibanum
Banana	Banana, Plantain Tea, Psyllium	Abaca, Manila Hemp, Plantain

* Submembers of the Rose family.

Botanical List of Food Families (cont.)

FAMILY	FOOD	RELATED PLANTS, EXTRACTS OR ALTERNATE IDENTIFICATION
Beech	Chestnut	Beech, Oak, Horse Chestnut (tree)
Water Chestnut	Ling Nut, Singhara Nut	
Chinese Water Chestnuts	Chinese Water Chestnuts	
Birch	Filbert, Hazelnut, Oil of Birch	Birch Tree
Borage	Borage, Comfrey Tea	Forget-me-not, Alkanet, Bugloss, Lungwort
Brazil Nut	Brazil Nut	Tree yields red dye
Buckthorn	Buckthorn Tea, Jujube (tree or shrub)	Buckthorn Syrup, Cascara Sagrada
Buckwheat	Buckwheat, Coccolaba, Rhubarb, Garden Sorrel	Knotweed
Buttercup		Aconite, Lenten Rose, Celandine, Buttercup, Clematis, Columbine, Delphinium, Larkspur, Monkshood, Peony, Hepatica
Cactus	Tequila, Prickly Pear	
Caper	Caper	
Carnation		Carnation, Pink, Sweet William
Cashew	Cashew, Mango, Pistachio	Poison Ivy, Poison Sumac
Chicle	Chicle Gum (from Sapodilla tree; also called Marmalade Plum tree)	

Botanical List of Food Families (cont.)

Citrus	Citric Acid, Citron, Citrange, Citranquequat, Grapefruit, Kumquat, Lemon, Lime, Limequat, Orange (Pumelo, Shaddock), Tangerine, Tangelo, Angostura Bitters	
Coca		Cocaine
Cola Nut	Chocolate, Cocoa, Cola Nut, Kutira Gum, Sterculia	Rope Fiber
Coffee	Coffee, Royoc, Indian Mulberry	
Composite	Globe Artichoke, Jerusalem Artichoke, Burdock, Camomile, Chicory, Dandelion, Endive, Escarole, Lettuce, Oyster Plant (vegetable oyster), Safflower Oil, Salsify, Cardoon, Sunflower Seed or Oil, Tarragon, Yarrow, Boneset Tea, Celtuse, Absinthe	Arnica, Aster, Bachelor's Button, Mum, Chamomile, Chrysanthemum, Cornflower, Dahlia, Daisy, Gaillardia (Blanket Flower), Gazonia (Treasure Flower), Heliopsis, Helipterum, Layia (Tidy Tip), Marigold, Pyrethrum, Ragweed, Sunflower, Zinnia, Cosmos, Blessed Thistle, Elecampane, Tansy, Lad's Love, Feverfew, Lavender Cotton, Wormwood, Cragweed, Sagebrush, Ironweed, Veronica
Curry Powder	Not one spice but a blend of spices	
Cycad	Kaffir bread	Cycas
Ebony	Date Plum, Persimmon	Ebony tree
Elm	Slippery Elm Tea	Chinese and Siberian Elm are resistant to Dutch Elm Disease

Botanical List of Food Families (cont.)

FAMILY	FOOD	RELATED PLANTS, EXTRACTS OR ALTERNATE IDENTIFICATION
Flacourtia	Kei Apple, Ceylon Gooseberry	
Foxglove		Digitalis, Figwort, Snapdragon, Verbascum (Purple Mullein)
Fungi	Moldy Cheeses, Mushroom, Yeast	Toadstools, Decaying Plants, Antibiotics
Garcinia	Mangosteen	
Gentian	Gentian Tea	Centaury
Geranium		Geranium, Nasturtium, Pelargonium
Ginger	Cardamom, Ginger, Turmeric	
Gooseberry	Currant (black, red, and white), Gooseberry	
Goosefoot	Beet, Beet Sugar, Spinach, Swiss Chard	Lamb's Quarters, Thistle, Kochia
Gourd (Melon)	Cantaloupe (muskmelon), Cocozelle, Cucumber, Casaba, Cassabanana, Curuba, Honeydew Melon, Spanish Melon, Persian Melon, Pumpkin, Squash (all varieties), Vegetable Marrow, Watermelon, Zucchini	
Grains	Barley (malt, whiskeys, ale, lager, some liqueurs), Cane Sugar (brown sugar, white sugar, molasses, rum),	Grass (all varieties), Citronella, Lemon Grass

Botanical List of Food Families (cont.)

Grape	Corn (cerulose, corn oil, corn starch, corn syrup, bourbon, dextrose, glucose), Millet, Oat, Rice (wild rice), Rye, Sorghum, Wheat (bran, gluten flour, durum, graham flour, wheat germ, cake flour, all-purpose flour), Bamboo Shoots, Pumpernickel
	Cream of Tartar, Grape, Raisin, Brandy, Port, Sherry, Wine, Champagne, Wine Vinegar, Vermouth
Heath	Blueberry, Cranberry, Dangleberry, Huckleberry, Uva-ursi, Wintergreen, Bearberry
	Azalea, Heather, Rhododendron
Heliotrope	Garden Heliotrope (Valeriana) used in medicine as Allheal or St. George's Herb
	Valerianella (Lamb's Lettuce or Corn Salad)
Honey	Honey, Bee Nectar, Beeswax
	Royal Jelly
Honeysuckle	Elderberry
	Honeysuckle
Hypericum	St. John's Wort Tea
Iris	Saffron
	Crocus, Gladiolus, Iris, Orris (used as a scent in cosmetics)
Laurel	Avocado, Bay Leaf, Camphor, Cinnamon, Laurel, Sassafras

Botanical List of Food Families (cont.)

FAMILY	FOOD	RELATED PLANTS, EXTRACTS OR ALTERNATE IDENTIFICATION
Legume	Acacia, Arabic, Kidney Bean, Green Bean, Lima Bean, Jack Bean, Navy Bean, Soy Bean (soya flour and oil), Wax Bean, Tonca Bean, Locust Bean Gum, Carob, Cassia, Fenugreek, Licorice, Lentil, Black-Eyed Pea, Chick Pea, Green Pea, Split Pea, Peanut (and oil), Karaya, Suakin, Talca Gum, Tamarind, Field Pea, Alfalfa, Indian Breadroot, Lucerne, St. John's Bread, Urd Flour, Mungo Bean, Tragacanth, Pinto Bean	Cassia (used in laxatives and cathartics), Mimosa, Milk Vetch, Clover, Senna (sometimes used in place of artificial cinnamon flavor), Lecithin (derived from soya)
Lily	Aloes, Asparagus, Chives, Garlic, Indian Cucumber Root, Leek, Onion, Sarsaparilla, Shallot	Lily (all varieties), Hyacinth, Trillium, Tulip, Yucca, Solomon's Seal, Adder's Tongue
Linden	Linden Tea	Basswood and Linden Trees
Linseed	Flax (flaxseed), Linseed	Linen
Litchi	Litchi nut	
Macadamia Nut	Macadamia Nut, Queensland Nut	Protea Plant produces a sugar
Mallow	Althea Root Tea, Cottonseed (Cottonseed Flour), Gumbo, Okra	Cotton, Hibiscus, Hollyhock
Maple	Maple Sugar and Syrup	Elder and Maple trees

Botanical List of Food Families (cont.)

May Apple		Podophyllin
Mint	Balm, Bergamot, Basil, Catnip, Chinese Artichoke, Horehound, Marjoram, Menthol, Mint, Peppermint, Rosemary, Sage, Savoury, Spearmint, Thyme, Pennyroyal Tea, Betony (Chinese Artichoke)	Lavender, Flowering Mint
Morning Glory	Sweet Potato, Yam	Morning Glory
Mulberry	Breadfruit, Fig, Mulberry, Hops	Rubber Plant
Mustard	Cabbage, Cauliflower, Celery Cabbage, Chinese Cabbage, Collard, Broccoli, Brussels Sprout, Horseradish, Radish, Kale, Sea Kale, Kohlrabi, Mustard, Mustard Greens, Rutabaga, Turnip, Garden Cress, Pepper Cress, Pepper Grass, Watercress, Colza, Sauerkraut	Heliophila, Mustard Seed
Myrtle	Allspice, Bayberry, Clove, Eucalyptus, Australian Brush Cherry, Guava, Rose Apple	Blue Gum, Kino
Nettle	Hop, Oregano	Nettle, Verbena, Hashish, Marijuana
New Zealand Spinach	New Zealand Spinach	Purslane

Botanical List of Food Families (cont.)

FAMILY	FOOD	RELATED PLANTS, EXTRACTS OR ALTERNATE IDENTIFICATION
Nightshade	Brinjal, Eggplant, Cayenne, Capsicum, Chili Pepper, Ground Cherry, Thorn Apple, Red Pepper, Banana Pepper, Bell Pepper, Green Pepper, Sweet Pepper, Paprika, Pimiento, Tabasco, Tomato, Potato	Tobacco, Belladonna, Nicotiana, Thorn Apple, Nicandra (Apple of Peru), Stramonium
Nutmeg	Mace, Nutmeg	
Olive	Black Olive, Green Olive, Ripe Olive, Olive Oil	Lilac, Privet, Jasmine
Orchid	True Vanilla, Gum Guaiacum	Orchids (all varieties)
Oxalis	Oxalis Tea (cure for scurvy)	
Palm	Coconut, Date, Sago	
Papaw	Papaya or Passion Fruit, Custard Apple, Alligator Apple, Pond Apple, Annona	Papain
Parsley	Angelica, Anise, Carrot, Celery, Celeriac, Celery Seed, Caraway Seed, Chervil, Sweet Cicely, Coriander, Comino, Cumin, Dill, Fennel, Ferula Gum, Gum Galbanum, Kummel, Lovage, Parsley, Parsnips, Samphire	Asafetida, Musk-root, Sumbul, Giant Fennel

Botanical List of Food Families (cont.)

Pepper	Black and White Pepper only
Pine or Cypress	Juniper, Pine Kernels, Piñon; Fir trees, Pine trees (all varieties), Sandarac Tree Resin, Turpentine
Pineapple	Pineapple
Plantain	Plantain Tea, Psyllium, Banana
Pomegranate	Pomegranate
Poppy	Poppy Seed and Oil; Argemone, Opium, all Poppies, Morphine, Heroin
Quinine	Cinchona
Ruta	Rutin Tea
Seaweed	Dulse, Kelp; Irish Moss, Carrageen
Sesame	Sesame Seed and Oil; Beni, Benne, Gingelly, Gingily, Teel or Til Oils
Styrax	Gum Benzoin or Benjamin
Tapioca	Castor Bean, Tapioca; Cascarilla, Cassava, Castor Oil, Chinese Tallow or Vegetable Tallow (candle wax)
Tea	Green Tea, Pekoe Tea
Violet	Pansy, Violet
Walnut	Butternut, Hickory Nut, Pecan, Black Walnut, English Walnut
Willow	Aspen, Cottonwood, Poplar trees, all Willows
Witch Hazel	Sweet Gum, Witch Hazel

Vegetable Gums The term *vegetable gum* encompasses members of twelve different botanical families. An allergy to one gum, therefore, does not necessarily mean that the person is allergic to all gums. He or she must find out which specific gum causes the allergic reaction.

Because vegetable gums are inexpensive, they are used extensively in commercial foods as fillers and binders. They also retard melting in frozen foods. Different gums have different properties, and each is used for its own individuality in different types of products.

Inhalation of dried flakes of vegetable gum can cause respiratory symptoms in a gum-sensitive person (for example, while combing hair after using setting lotion containing gum). Eating the gum can cause any type of allergic reaction.

Cheseborough-Pond's, a major cosmetic manufacturer, advises that when natural gums are used, a preservative, germicide, or fungicide must be added to the product to prevent deterioration of the gum. For this reason, synthetic gums are replacing natural gums in order to achieve longer shelf life for cosmetics.

Some manufacturers of surgical tape use acrylic resin adhesive, and others use synthetic rubber and resin mixture.

Table 8.3. Vegetable Gums

GUM	FAMILY	USES
Acacia (mimosa)	Legume	Perfume, tanning, timber
Arabic	Legume	Dyeing, fruit drinks, mucilage, printing
Suakin	Legume	
Talca	Legume	
Karaya	Legume	Mucilage, pharmaceuticals, straw hats, textile stiffener
Tragacanth	Legume	Same as karaya

Carob (Locust Bean)	Legume	Chocolate substitute
Ammoniacum	Ammoniacum	Cement, medicinal stimulant (spirits of ammonia)
Gum Benjamin (Gum Benzoin)	Styrax	Incense, medicinal use in expectorants, inhalants, and external antiseptics, scent of vanilla in lotions, toilet water, tooth powders
Chicle	Chicle	Chewing gum
Eucalyptus	Myrtle	Aromatic spirits, kine resin, tannin, timber
Ferula (Fennel), also called Asafetida, Muskroot, or Sumbul	Parsley	Antispasmodic, stimulant
Galbanum	Parsley	Same as ferula
Guaiacum	Orchid	
Irish Moss	Seaweed or dried and bleached	Cosmetics, laxative, toothpaste
Carrageen (carragheenan)	Extract of Irish moss	
Kutira	Cola Nut or Mallow	One variety for rope, Chinese variety for drinks, jellies
Olibanum	Balsam	Frankincense
Quince	Rose (submember)	Pectin
Sweet Gum	Witch Hazel	Astringent, medicinally for chest complaints, sedative, tonic, skin diseases, perfume, timber

When will an offending food provoke an allergic reaction?

Allergic people react to an allergic food when they have reached their allergy threshold. Thus, those with a very low allergy threshold may react when they merely smell the food allergen, whereas those with a very high threshhold may be able to eat substantial amounts of the offending food without experiencing any reaction at all.

Factors that may operate, separately or together, to produce allergic symptoms or to bring a person to his or her allergy threshold include:

> Simultaneous eating of two or more allergenic foods
> Fatigue
> Infection
> Simultaneous contact with two or more allergens
>> (for example, eating an allergenic substance while near an allergenic animal)
> Seasonal airborne allergies
> Sensitivity to certain weather conditions
> Excessive eating at one sitting
> Excessive consumption of alcohol
> Over- or undercooking of food (for example, boiled milk may be tolerated, but not whole milk from the container).

What are some of the other factors involved in the diagnosis of a food allergy?

Food contaminants, including pesticides, may be present in certain foods and can be misleading when one is evaluating allergic reactions. Thus, patients who drink milk that contains penicillin—used to treat cow udder infections—and who are allergic to the drug, develop an allergic reaction to the drug and not to the food, though the latter may appear to be the allergen. On occasion, a fish allergy may be mistaken for a milk allergy; milk may contain traces of fish protein present in cow feed.

What role do food additives play in food allergy?

Until the last few years, food additives were considered safe, or at least insignificant in normal doses. Today, such additives are suspected of being responsible for reactions similar to those attributed to food allergy. Additives are synthetic chemicals that add color, taste, and texture to such foods as candies, gelatin desserts, mustard, and canned goods. Unfortunately, because some additives are used so widely and labeled inaccurately, it is often difficult to avoid them.

A reaction to food additives is probably not caused by allergies, but rather by a toxic reaction to some substance in the additive. (It is sometimes claimed that food additives are responsible for some psychoneurotic and hyperactive behavior in children.) Hives, asthma, rhinitis, and constipation are a few of the possible reactions to additives that may seem to be caused (as they often are) by a food allergy.

What is the most effective treatment of food allergy?
Once the offending foods have been discovered, the most effective treatment is simply to eliminate them from the diet.

Do I need a doctor's advice to devise a food allergy diet?
All food allergy diets *must* be prescribed and checked by a doctor. Otherwise, an allergy patient may unknowingly impair his or her health by failing to substitute a nutritionally equivalent food for the offending food. Doctors can plan a well-balanced, nutritious diet using safe substitutes and, perhaps, adding vitamins and minerals. Or, they can suggest others, such as dieticians, who can provide such counseling.

Can allergenic foods eventually be restored to the diet without causing allergic symptoms?
After you have avoided the offending foods for at least six months, you may, if your doctor approves, try a *small amount* of the food. If the symptoms do not recur, you may be able to take a little of the food on occasion.

People experiencing severe immediate reactions to certain foods, such as eggs, shellfish, nuts, buckwheat, or mustard, often will do so for the rest of their lives. *No food causing severe allergic symptoms should ever be eaten at any time, in any amount.* This requires extreme diligence and scrutiny on the part of the patient, particularly when dining away from home. Tasting only a tiny amount of the food before considering it safe to eat is a good habit to get into in this type of situation. Even this, however, is not always totally safe. Because the content of a food cannot always be known ahead of time, allergy patients who must eat away from home should carry Adrenalin or another prescribed drug if an allergic food is inadvertently eaten.

What can be done if the specific food causing an allergenic reaction cannot be determined?
When the exact cause of the food allergy remains unknown after all diagnostic tests have been completed, your doctor may prescribe

drugs to alleviate the symptoms. (Unfortunately, such drugs cannot cure the allergy itself.) Another approach is the rotary diet, in which no food is repeated within a five-day span, thus reducing symptoms.

Is it possible to have a food allergy and still lead a normal life?
Once one has been diagnosed as having a particular food allergy, life is not over. On the contrary, a new life can begin when one knows the foods that are safe to eat—and the ones that are not.

Food Allergy Cooking

What kind of diet should be followed if one is allergic to milk?
The only way to deal effectively with milk allergy is to avoid milk and all milk products systematically until all symptoms (including hives, rhinitis, eczema, asthma, vomiting, diarrhea, gas, constipation, and anaphylactic shock) are controlled or have disappeared. According to allergists, such reactions are variously caused by lactalbumin (a simple protein), milk sugar, and casein (another protein), all of which are found in milk.

The first step in avoiding foods that contain milk is to learn how to read carefully and to comprehend the ingredient labels of prepared foods. *When no ingredients are listed, the food should not be eaten under any circumstances.* This also applies when ingredient labels indicate that the product contains any of the following: milk (whole, skim, evaporated, condensed, or dried), cream, milk solids, yogurt, butter, margarine, whey, cheese, buttermilk, sour cream, lactose, caseinate, lactalbumin lactate, and sodium caseinate. A simple rule of thumb regarding any substance you are not sure about is: When in doubt, don't.

The following prepared foods may contain milk, and their ingredient labels should be checked carefully before you purchase and eat them:

> Breaded meats and fish
> Creamed soups and sauces
> Milk chocolate, chocolate creams, and candy bars
> Gravies and sauces
> Margarines
> Processed meat such as hot dogs (milk is used as a binder or
>   filler)

Baked goods (cakes, pancakes, cookies, bread, cream pies, and so on)

Desserts (puddings, ice cream, sherbet, junket, and so on)

Although this list may at first seem overwhelming, replacing milk is actually quite simple. For cow's milk a variety of products can be substituted, including Ener-G-Foods' Soyquik (lactose- and gluten-free), Soyagen (for adults; lactose-free), and Soyalac (for infants; lactose-free). These are all made from the soy plant, which is tolerated by most people. (A teaspoon of lime juice per cup, or molasses, honey, or vanilla extract, may be used to improve the flavor.) Other possible milk substitutes include Nutramagen, a lactose-free formula with a protein base, and Gerber's Meat-Base Formula (MBF) for babies. Nondairy creamer (if it is casein-free) can be used instead of milk in coffee. You can also use goat's milk, or even plain water. When making hot cereal, for instance, just use a little more water than usual and add a little zest to the taste with brown sugar, honey, or molasses. Omelets and scrambled eggs are light and fluffy when water is used as a substitute.

Replacing butter does not present any major problem, either; it can be replaced by any one of a number of milk-free margarines available. You may be able to replace cheese with goat's milk cheese, with soybean tofu cheese, or with Fisher's Chees-ola (which contains milk products but is low in lactose). Check with your doctor before using any of these substitute products.

When cooking, use oil rather than animal fat; on salads, use an oil-and-vinegar dressing. If you dislike margarine, toast your bread and spread jam or honey on it while it is still hot. Excellent sandwiches can be made with ketchup, mustard, mayonnaise, barbecue sauce, and relish.

Whipped cream can be replaced by nondairy dessert toppings, and when such recipes as that for beef stroganoff call for sour cream, prepare this mixture: for 1 cup of imitation sour cream, stir 4 tablespoons of allowed starch into ¾ cup water and ¼ cup vinegar; adjust these proportions as necessary to suit the recipe and your taste.

Whenever a food is being substituted, remember to compensate for the lost nutritious ingredients by incorporating the necessary vitamins and minerals into your diet. If you are allergic to milk, you can provide your body with calcium, for example, in the form of dolomite powder tablets or bone meal. The protein ordinarily obtained from milk can also be found in such other foods as eggs, meat, fish, whole grains, peas, vegetables, and fruit.

Once again, be sure to check with your doctor before planning to incorporate any of the above-mentioned substitutes, dietary supplements, and foods into your diet. Your specific type of milk allergy may not tolerate certain products.

What kind of diet should egg-sensitive people follow?

Egg allergy is less common than milk allergy, but the allergic threshold is much lower. Sometimes, merely touching or smelling an egg can produce symptoms. This also happens when one is given vaccines for measles, mumps, rubella, and flu, all of which vaccines are made with eggs.

Any egg, be it chicken, goose, duck, or turkey, can produce symptoms if you have an egg allergy. The avoidance list also includes eggs in any form, fresh, dried, or powdered, as well as yolk and albumin. Candy is often brushed with egg white for luster, and pies are, too, so that they bake to a golden brown. Coffee and homemade beer, as well as some soups, may be clarified with egg shells. Generally speaking, you should beware of such foods as waffles, cakes, pastries, ice cream, and sherbet (unless made from an egg-free powder), creamy salad dressings and mayonnaise, heavy sauces, bouillon and broths, root beer, Ovaltine and Ovomalt, meat loaf and sausages, noodles, and baking products.

Egg-free meals can be prepared in a variety of ways. Ener-G-Foods' Egg Replacer (formerly Jolly Joan) is one of the most readily available egg substitutes. You can also replace one egg by mixing 2 tablespoons of flour, ½ teaspoon of shortening, ½ teaspoon of baking powder, and 2 tablespoons of liquid. A package of Knox gelatin or a mashed banana can be used as a binder for each missing egg. Not all cake mixes absolutely require eggs. If you wish, you may write to the company making a particular recipe and ask for information.

Many so-called egg substitutes available today are not egg-free, as they contain egg whites, the major source of egg allergen for most people.

Remember to eat plenty of meat, fish, poultry, liver, cheese, dried beans, or nuts to get the amount of protein and B vitamins usually derived from eggs.

What if I am allergic to wheat?

If you or your child is allergic to wheat, learn to avoid the following ingredients: flour; wheat flour; wheat starch; gluten flour; graham flour; cracked wheat flour; enriched flour; monosodium glutamate (MSG); hydrolyzed vegetable protein (HVP); whole wheat flour;

wheat germ; bran, cake, and pastry flour; and durum wheat.

Foods to be eliminated absolutely include biscuits, breads, and bread crumbs; candy of unknown composition; breaded products (for example, fish, poultry, and meat); malted milk, beer, ale, wine, and instant coffee containing wheat flour; luncheon meats, hamburgers, hot dogs, and sausages (unless they are pure meat); cheese sauces and spreads (unless they are wheat-free); noodles (unless made with potato or rice flour); potato dishes containing wheat flour; and certain canned soups. Sometimes liquor, which is usually made from wheat, cannot be tolerated in any form. Be careful with items labeled "starch"—they may have wheat starch. Avoid medication, such as vitamins, that may contain wheat, as well as patent medicines whose labels do not identify ingredients. Always check with your physician or pharmacist before having a prescription filled or purchasing medicine.

Wheat can be replaced by products such as Ener-G-Foods' rice baking mix and barley mix, as well as by tapioca, sago, rice, potato, soya, corn, arrowroot, buckwheat, rye, oats, or barley. Chinese grocery stores sell noodles in all shapes and sizes made from rice flour. Many patients are able to tolerate 100-percent sour-rye bread, which is sometimes available at specialty food stores. (Be sure it contains no wheat flour.) The following substitutions can replace one cup of wheat flour:

½ cup barley flour
1¼ cups rye flour
1 cup rye meal
1⅓ cup ground rolled oats
½ cup rye flour and ½ cup potato flour
⅔ cup rye flour and ⅓ cup potato flour
⅝ cup rice flour and ⅓ cup rye flour

What kind of diet should gluten-sensitive people follow?

Gluten is the elastic rubbery protein that binds the dough in such foods as bread, biscuits, cakes, and pastry. Allergy to gluten requires avoidance of wheat and rye, possibly barley and oats, as well as of all gluten-containing foods. The last group includes flour, wheat flour, gluten flour, graham flour, cracked wheat flour, enriched flour, malt, malt syrup, oatmeal, oats, rye, rye flour, barley, barley flour, monosodium glutamate (MSG), hydrolyzed vegetable protein (HVP), durum flour, dried peas or beans, and millet.

Wheat starch is the traditional substitute for gluten-free baking, but it is not totally gluten-free. If this is tolerated, Aproten Pasta made by Henkel Corporation can be used as a pasta substitute. Sago, tapioca, rice, potato, soya, corn, arrowroot, buckwheat, and soft wheat (cake and pastry flour) are additional cooking substitutes. Ener-G-Foods' Rice Bread and Nutine (gluten- and wheat-free) are two ready-made gluten-free breads. If you make your own bread, try using a combination of several allowed flours. (See the baking tips given below in this chapter.)

The following flour-and-meal combination can be used as a substitute in gluten-free diets. It requires at least five or six siftings and long, slow baking:

1 cup corn flour
¾ cup coarse corn meal
1 scant cup of fine corn meal
⅞ cup rice flour
⅝ cup rice flour and ⅓ cup potato flour

1 cup soy flour and ¾ cup potato flour
⅝ cup potato flour (sometimes called potato starch)
1 scant cup wheat starch

The following gluten-free flour mix should be thoroughly blended and can be used in any recipe calling for all-purpose flour except for bread, gingerbread, doughnuts, fritters, and shortbread. It also requires at least five or six siftings and long, slow baking:

2 cups wheat starch
¾ cup corn flour
¾ cup potato flour
¼ cup soya flour

1 cup rice flour
6 tablespoons arrowroot flour
6 tablespoons tapioca flour

What about corn allergy and corn-free diets?

If you are allergic to corn, you must avoid eating and sometimes even smelling corn and all corn-related products. Some items to be avoided are: cornflakes, baking powder, corn oil, corn syrup, corn flour, corn sugar, fritters, cerelose, sorbitol, dyno, cartose, cornstarch, chewing gum, soya milk, powdered sugar, caramel coloring, dextrose, white vinegar, commercially canned jam and preserves, fruit canned in syrup, some substitute egg yolks, and aspirin and other tablets. You should also beware of such adhesive gums as those on stamps, envelopes, and tapes, since they contain small quantities of corn. Any medication with gluconate contains corn.

Cornstarch can be replaced by Featherweight cornstarch. You can also make your own corn-free baking powder by substituting the following mixture in any recipe:

1 part baking soda
1 part cream of tartar

1 part potato starch

Or, you can pulverize and mix the following:

1 ounce cream of tartar	½ ounce tartaric acid
5 ounces bicarbonate of soda	4 ounces flour

For heavy batters such as Christmas cake, try using equal amounts of cream of tartar and baking soda.

What are some simple baking hints that come in handy when one is baking allergy-free recipes?

Although you may think otherwise, allergy-free baking is not very different from your regular baking methods. The following information will help guide you.

Heavier flour and yeast-free baked products have a heavier texture, and their taste depends on your choice of flour. If you use dark-colored baking pans, especially the black-finish kind, turn the oven temperature 25 degrees F lower than the recipe calls for. When baking cookies, set your timer for two or three minutes less than the time the recipe calls for. Your cookie sheets and your oven influence baking time. Watch the bottom sheet carefully when baking two sheets at a time.

When using dark-finish pans for breads and cakes, set the timer for as much as ten minutes less than the time indicated on the recipe and check the progress frequently, without opening the oven door. For future reference, mark the appropriate time on the recipe.

The weather is another important factor in baking results. Since flours can lose moisture in the winter, some recipes may require the addition of liquid. If the dough is too soft to handle, add more flour. Sifting is not necessary before measuring. After combining the dry ingredients, however, sifting will ensure that the ingredients do not ball during mixing. If you are using a food processor, sifting is not necessary, since balling doesn't affect the final outcome, but do stir the flour before measuring. (The baking tips in this answer courtesy of Carol Rudoff, President, American Allergy Association, and Editor, *Living with Allergies*.)

Can a person be allergic to fruit?

Harmless though they may seem, some fruits may cause very unpleasant reactions in allergy-sensitive people. Strawberries and raspberries can provoke hives. Citrus fruit, including oranges, lemons, grapefruits, tangerines, and limes, may cause reactions affecting the chest and nose. Abdominal pain and throat irritation may occur after eating such fruits as peaches, apples, watermelon, cherries, and bananas.

When determining the specific nature of the fruit allergy, two factors must be considered. First, if you are sensitive to one kind of fruit, it must be established whether or not you are also allergic to other members of the particular food family. (See, in this regard, the Botanical List of Food Families above in this chapter.)

An allergic reaction to fruit may depend on whether the fruit is ripe, peeled, canned, cooked, or frozen. Someone who reacts to a particular fresh fruit may not do so if it is eaten cooked, and vice versa.

What are the dietary restrictions and options if one is allergic to poultry, to meat, or to fish?

If you are allergic to one member of the poultry group, such as turkey, all members, including chicken, goose, and squab, are forbidden. The allergy may not stem from the poultry itself, however, but from the eggs it sometimes contains or from the hormones and antibiotics frequently added to the fowl's meal. In this case, capon is often tolerated.

If you are allergic to one kind of fish, caution is advised in eating any other kind. If you are allergic to one kind of shellfish, avoidance of all shellfish is advised. People reactive to fish, however, can often tolerate shellfish and vice versa.

If you are allergic to meat, including beef, veal, pork, ham, and bacon, avoid as well any meat-containing products such as gelatin and extracts made from cow and calf organs. Also to be avoided are lard and bacon drippings found, respectively, in cake shortening and fried foods. All-vegetable shortenings are safe.

The best meat "substitutes" are the less allergenic meats of lamb and mutton. Ground lamb can be used quite successfully to make hamburgers and in such recipes calling for ground meat as those for shepherd's pie and meatloaf. If you do not have your own grinder, ask your butcher to do the grinding for you. Have the butcher first put through the grinder a bit of lamb fat to remove all traces of any previously ground meat. Additional possibilities that can add variety to the menu are ground lamb livers and kidneys. For instance, one kidney and liver ground and mixed into ten pounds of ground lamb add nutritious flavor to the lamb.

What are some of the other food allergies and what are the dietary restrictions involved?

The most frequently encountered food allergies have already been discussed. As stated previously, however, one can be or become allergic to almost any food, including spices and herbs, chocolate, beverages, and/or nuts.

Allergy to spices and herbs can be controlled by simply eliminating the spices and herbs in question and any products containing them. Sensitivity to chocolate usually provokes abdominal pain and migraine headaches; if such sensitivity is present, chocolate should be avoided, as well as cocoa butter and cola beverages. Substitute carob powder in any recipes calling for chocolate. One square of baking chocolate is equivalent to one to three tablespoons of carob powder, plus either one-half tablespoon of margarine or two tablespoons of water.

Some people are allergic to coffee as well as to such coffee substitutes as chicory, chestnuts, cereals, and peas. All products containing coffee, such as coffee ice cream, coffee yogurt, coffee candy, coffee beverages, and some coffee-containing medicines, should be eliminated from the diet.

Other allergies, such as those to nuts and peanuts, can be treated effectively simply by consulting the Botanical List of Food Families chart above and then avoiding all the related foods listed.

What are some simple tips that can help turn the allergen-free diet from an ordeal into a pleasure?

This question is of most concern to the parent of the allergic child. As stated previously, she should try to serve as many nonallergenic meals as possible that can be eaten by the entire family. She should be on the lookout for recipes that do not use the allergenic food or that require so little of it that substitution is easy. When recipes can be prepared almost to completion without the allergenic food, she should just eliminate the allergenic ingredient from the child's meal. Thus, for example, if the parent is making beef stroganoff, she should serve it without the sour cream to her milk-sensitive child and with the sour cream to the other members of her family. The more the allergic child's food resembles the family food, the happier and more cooperative the child will be.

Solutions to the problem of feeding the allergic child may be found beyond the traditional limits of Western cooking. Two excellent sources of nonallergenic dishes are the cuisines of China and the East Indies, where the ingredients common in North American and European cooking are rarely used. Challenging as this may seem, one's efforts may be well rewarded by the child's pleasure in experiencing simultaneously an exotic cuisine and relief from allergy symptoms.

Lunches can be a problem for the parent of an allergic child and may require some creativity. The following tips will undoubtedly make life easier:

Instead of trying to make a sandwich with gluten-free bread

(purchased or homemade) that may not taste like the real thing, the parent of a gluten-sensitive child can pack a lunch including a slice of gluten-free bread buttered with margarine, a salad, a hard-boiled egg, and some fruit.

Banana bread is a satisfying substitute for the gluten-sensitive child. This can be made by mashing three small or large bananas into the wet ingredients for four loaves of bread, with a little sugar if desired. Taco shells or pita bread pouches stuffed with cold meat, lettuce, tomatoes, and cheese make a more than adequate sandwich substitute for people on the gluten-free diet.

Homemade soups, stews, and casseroles stored in wide-necked Thermos jars, plus a piece of fruit, make for a nutritious, healthy, and tasty lunch.

Whether it be breakfast, lunch, or dinner, and regardless of the diet in question, variety and creativity are the key words. Vegetables, meat, bread, fruit, and beverages should be as varied as possible. Meals can be brightened up with colorful napkins or with a favorite snack item, such as figs, allowed on the child's particular diet. If birthday cakes are not allowed, a brick of ice cream topped with chocolate fudge sauce and whipped cream can, if no allergies forbid, make an excellent substitute.

It is up to the parent to make meals as pleasant as possible and thus to instill a cooperative attitude in the child. Thus, younger allergic children should not be nagged, hurried, or scolded at the table. Family conversation should, whenever possible, be steered away from the subject of food and table manners. Once the child is psychologically in control of his problem and enjoys his meals, parents can start correcting any undesirable aspects of his behavior.

If the child rejects a meal, this should be accepted quietly. However, he should not be allowed to eat anything until the next meal. It is easier to ensure a nutritionally sound diet through meals than through snacking.

A most important, and possibly most difficult step involves receiving cooperation from others. This is particularly hard in the case of a child. Friends, relatives, and neighbors must be told kindly but firmly not to give the child *any* of the forbidden foods. Most hosts and hostesses will gladly inform the parent of a food-allergic child about the menu they are planning so that parents can match the child's special food with the food to be served.

By the same token, the child has to learn early on to reject certain foods independently. Once the taste is lost for the forbidden food, once it is grasped that eating any of it will make him or her feel unwell, the task should become a good deal easier.

What are some appetizing yet simple allergy-free recipes suitable for the entire family?

The number of allergy-free recipes that can be enjoyed by all members of the family is enormous. The following recipes, courtesy of the Allergy Information Association, Weston, Ontario, Canada, suggest the variety of allergy-free recipes readily available for soups, entrées, vegetables, sauces, and salad dressings.

Soups
(egg-free, gluten-free, wheat-free)

Potato Soup

5 cups sliced raw potato
½ cup finely chopped celery
1 tablespoon (or more) minced
    onion
1 medium carrot, grated
Salt and pepper to taste

Barely cover the mixture with water and simmer until potatoes are well cooked (about 10 minutes). Mash in own liquid, and add 1 tablespoon butter and enough milk to give desired consistency. Reheat and serve immediately. Makes 1–2 adult servings.

Tomato Bisque

1 28-ounce can tomatoes
½ onion, sliced
1 bay leaf
2 cups milk
1 beef bouillon cube
1 teaspoon sugar
¼ teaspoon nutmeg, if desired
½ cup dry (diet) bread crumbs
2 tablespoons butter
Few grains of pepper
Salt to taste

Combine tomatoes, onion, and bay leaf. Simmer for 10 minutes and press through a sieve. Slowly stir in milk and add bouillon cube dissolved in a small amount of the hot mixture. Add seasonings. Stir while heating. Do *not* boil. Add crumbs and butter. Serves 6.

Cream of Pea Soup

1 tablespoon margarine
1 tablespoon gluten-free flour (or
    ¼ cup infant rice cereal)
1 cup milk
1 jar strained peas
Salt to taste

Melt margarine. Stir in flour or cereal. Add milk and stir until sauce thickens. Fold in peas and add salt. Bring to a boil and serve. Serves 1.

Entrées
(egg-free, gluten-free, milk-free, wheat-free)

Beef Casserole

1½ pounds ground chuck beef
¾ pound sliced mushrooms (or one 10-ounce can)
1 green pepper, chopped
1 cup chopped celery
1 package dried onion soup mix
1 teaspoon Worcestershire sauce
6 ounces fine noodles (use rice vermicelli for gluten-free diets)

Grated cheese (omit for milk-free diets)
½ teaspoon salt
Pinch of thyme
1 28-ounce can tomatoes

Sauté beef, mushrooms, green pepper, and celery in oil. Add tomatoes, onion soup mix, Worcestershire sauce, salt, and thyme. Cook until excess moisture is gone. Cook rice noodles or vermicelli, drain well, and add to meat mixture. Put in casserole, adding grated cheese if allowed. Heat in 350° F oven for ½ to ¾ hour. If desired, omit mushrooms, celery, and tomatoes and substitute stuffed olives, canned corn niblets, and your favorite soup. Serves 12.

Shepherd's Meat Loaf
(*not* egg-free)

1 pound ground chuck beef
2 tablespoons diced onion
1 teaspoon salt
1 hot cooked medium potato, mashed (no milk)

½ teaspoon garlic powder
1 egg
½ pound fresh mushrooms, sliced
Ketchup

In an 8-inch square pan, thoroughly mix together meat, onion, salt, potato, garlic powder, and egg, and form a loaf of about 7 inches × 1½ inches. Firmly press mushroom slices over entire surface of loaf. Bake in 350° F oven for about 1 hour. Slice and serve with ketchup. Serves 3.

Jambalaya

2 slices chopped bacon
2 tablespoons chopped onion
2 cups tomatoes
1 cup water
Grated Parmesan or Cheddar cheese to taste (omit for milk-free diet)

¼ teaspoon salt
¼ teaspoon pepper
¾ cup uncooked rice
2 cups diced cooked ham, chicken, or turkey

Cook bacon slowly. Add onion, and cook until clear. Add tomatoes, water, and seasonings. Bring to a boil. Add rice and boiling liquid, gently stirring with fork until the mixture comes to a boil. Cover tightly, reduce heat, and let simmer for 20 minutes. Fold in the diced meat when rice is tender and dry. Heat to serving temperature and add cheese if allowed. Serves 4.

Lamb Stew

½ pound lamb, cut for stew
1 tablespoon rice flour
¾ teaspoon salt
1¼ cups hot water

1½ cups diced, pared sweet
  potatoes
1 tablespoon lamb drippings

Roll lamb in mixture of flour and salt. Brown in hot drippings. Add water, cover, and simmer for 1 hour. Add potatoes, cover, and cook for 25 minutes or longer, or until tender. Prepare gravy with liquid and 1 tablespoon flour. Serves 3.

Lamb Liver Slices with Spiced Prune Sauce

⅔ cup dried prunes
1½ cups water
¼ cup sugar
½ teaspoon citric acid crystals

1 pound sliced lamb liver
1 teaspoon salt
2 tablespoons lamb drippings
1 tablespoon rice flour

Cover and simmer prunes in water until tender. Drain and cut up prunes, reserving liquid.

Combine sugar, citric acid crystals, and rice flour. Gradually stir in liquid from prunes (about ½ cup). Cook and stir until slightly thickened. Add cut-up prunes and heat thoroughly. Sprinkle liver with salt. Brown on both sides in lamb drippings (about 2 minutes on each side). Serve with prune sauce. Serves 3.

Tuna Soufflé
(*not* egg-free)

3 tablespoons shortening
2 tablespoons diced green pepper
2 tablespoons minced onion
1 cup water
2½ tablespoons rice flour

1 teaspoon salt
1 tablespoon lemon juice
1 5½- or 7-ounce can tuna,
  drained and flaked
4 eggs, separated

In medium-size saucepan, melt shortening over low heat; in it, sauté green pepper and onion for about 5 minutes. Stir in rice flour; cook, stirring, for about 1 minute. Add water and cook, stirring constantly until mixture thickens. Stir in salt, lemon juice, and tuna. Add egg yolks and blend well. In a large bowl, beat egg whites until stiff but not dry. Carefully fold in tuna mixture, then pour into ungreased 1½-quart casserole or soufflé dish. Bake in 350° F oven for about 1 hour. Serve immediately. Serves 4.

Salmon Bake
(*not* egg-free)

1½ cups precooked rice
1½ cups boiling water
1 7½-ounce can salmon,
   drained and flaked
2 teaspoons salt
¼ teaspoon black pepper

2 tablespoons minced onion
2 egg whites
1 egg
2 tablespoons melted milk-free
   margarine

Add rice to boiling water; cover; remove from heat; let stand for five minutes. Set oven temperature at 375° F. Combine salmon, rice, salt, pepper, and onion. Beat egg whites and egg; fold into salmon mixture and blend well. Press into buttered 8-inch square baking dish or loaf pan. Brush top with melted milk-free margarine. Bake in 375° F oven for 30 minutes or until firm and golden. Garnish with lemon wedges and parsley. Serves 4.

Pizza Rice Pie
(*not* egg-free)

2⅔ cups cooked rice
½ cup minced onion
2 eggs, beaten
3 tablespoons butter (or butter
   substitute for milk-free diets)
1 8-ounce can tomato sauce
¼ teaspoon oregano

¼ teaspoon basil
1 cup shredded mozzarella
   cheese (omit for milk-free
   diets)
4½ ounces pepperoni
¼ cup stuffed olives

Mix together rice, onion, eggs, and melted butter. Line 12-inch pizza pan with rice mixture. Bake for 12 minutes or until brown. Spread tomato sauce over rice crust. Sprinkle with oregano, basil, and shredded cheese. Top with pepperoni and olives. Bake at 350° F for 20 minutes. Let stand for a few minutes before serving after removing from oven. Serves 4.

Vegetables

Creamed Vegetable Casserole
(egg-free, gluten-free, wheat-free)

Green beans or carrots may be used as a substitute. If allergic to citrus, omit lemon juice and replace with $\frac{1}{16}$ teaspoon nutmeg.

1 10-ounce package frozen asparagus or broccoli	1 tablespoon lemon juice
1 cup skim milk	2 tablespoons fine diet bread crumbs
¼ teaspoon salt	½ teaspoon vegetable oil
2 tablespoons cream of rice cereal	paprika

Cook vegetable according to package directions. Drain. Combine skim milk and salt and heat over very low flame. Sprinkle in cream of rice cereal and cook, stirring constantly, for 1 minute. Remove from heat, cover, and let stand 4 minutes. Add lemon juice and beat well. Transfer vegetable to a greased baking dish and pour milk mixture over this. Mix gently with a fork. Combine bread crumbs with oil and sprinkle over vegetable. Add a few shakes of paprika. Bake at 375° F for about 20 minutes. Serves 4.

Potato Soufflé
(gluten-free, milk-free, wheat-free)

1½ cups instant mashed potatoes	1 7½-ounce can crab, or 1 cup diced roast meat, or 2 cups shredded Cheddar cheese (not for milk-free diets)
2¼ cups boiling water	
1 tablespoon milk-free margarine	
½ teaspoon salt	Dash of cayenne
4 eggs, separated	

Prepare mashed potatoes as directed, substituting water for milk. Slowly add beaten egg yolks to potatoes. Add crab and cayenne. Beat egg whites until stiff and then fold into potato mixture. Put in soufflé dish or 1½-quart casserole. Bake in 350° F oven for 50 minutes or until golden brown. Serves 6.

Spicy Mashed Potatoes
(gluten-free, milk-free, egg-free, wheat-free)

2 cups mashed potatoes, seasoned (do not add milk)	1 tablespoon chopped parsley
	2 tablespoons chopped onion
2 slices bacon, diced and cooked	2 tablespoons milk-free margarine

Combine all ingredients and serve at once. Serves 4.

Sauces
(gluten-free, milk-free, egg-free, wheat-free)

Tomato Sauce

2½ cups canned tomatoes
2 stalks celery, diced
1 small onion, diced

2 tablespoons ketchup
1 tablespoon brown sugar
1 tablespoon vinegar

Add celery and onions to tomatoes and simmer for 10 minutes. Fold in ketchup, brown sugar, and vinegar. Simmer until vegetables are cooked. (This mixture may be thickened with a gluten-free flour if desired.)

Spaghetti Sauce

¼ cup milk-free margarine
1 garlic clove, minced
¼ cup oil

2 cups mushrooms, sliced thin
¼ teaspoon oregano
   salt and pepper

Melt oil and milk-free margarine in frying pan, then add garlic and mushrooms. Fry until tender, stirring often. Add spices.

White Sauce

1 tablespoon milk-free
   margarine
1½ teaspoons potato starch (or any
   other gluten-free flour)

¼ teaspoon salt
½ cup soybean milk
1 teaspoon dried parsley
   (optional)

Melt milk-free margarine in saucepan. Add potato starch or gluten-free flour and salt and stir until well mixed. Add soybean milk and parsley and continue stirring until mixture thickens.

Hot Barbecue Sauce

2 teaspoons hot-pepper sauce
2½ cups chili sauce
1 teaspoon chili pepper
¾ cup oil
½ cup lemon juice

2 tablespoons tarragon vinegar
1 tablespoon brown sugar
1 bay leaf
1 teaspoon mustard
1 teaspoon salt

Combine ingredients and simmer for 15 minutes.

Sweet and Sour Sauce
(egg-free only)

1 can tomato soup
⅓ cup sugar

¼ cup vinegar

Boil vinegar. Add sugar, salt, cornstarch, and mustard to beaten eggs. ing time. This sauce can also be used cold as a salad dressing; hot on pork and beans (mix in and refrigerate for a day, covered); hot as a barbecue sauce.
NOTE: the quantities of sugar and vinegar can be adjusted to individual taste.

Salad Dressings

Creamy Salad Dressing
(*not* egg-free)

1 cup vinegar
1 heaping tablespoon cornstarch
1 teaspoon salt

⅔ cup sugar
2 eggs
1 teaspoon mustard

Boil vinegar. Add sugar, salt, cornstarch and mustard to beaten eggs. Combine a little hot vinegar to the egg mixture. Add egg mixture to the vinegar and bring to a full boil.

Macaroni or Potato Dressing
(egg-free, milk-free)

3 tablespoons flour
3 tablespoons sugar
1 teaspoon thyme
1 teaspoon salt

¾ cup Rich's Coffee Rich
¾ cup water
¼ cup vinegar

Mix dry ingredients in pan. Add Coffee Rich and water gradually, and stir until thick. Add vinegar and mix well.

Potato Flour Mayonnaise
(egg-free, gluten-free, milk-free, wheat-free)

1½ tablespoons potato flour
¼ teaspoon dry mustard
½ teaspoon salt
 2 teaspoons sugar
¼ cup cold water

¾ cup boiling water
 2 tablespoons lemon juice
 1 tablespoon white vinegar
½ cup salad oil
  Salt and pepper to taste

Mix dry ingredients in saucepan, then stir in cold water and mix well. Add hot water and cook just until mixture is clear. Let cool to lukewarm, then gradually add remaining ingredients, beating constantly.

Thousand Island Dressing
(egg-free, gluten-free, milk-free, wheat-free)

1 cup mayonnaise (your own
    diet preference)
4 tablespoons chili sauce
1 tablespoon chives (or onion)
3 tablespoons ketchup

1 teaspoon vinegar (or pickle juice
    if suited to diet)
2 tablespoons chopped red pepper
1 teaspoon paprika

Mix ingredients well and chill in refrigerator.

Paprika Salad Dressing
(egg-free, milk-free)

1 cup sugar
2 tablespoons flour
2 teaspoons thyme
1 tablespoon paprika

½ cup vinegar
½ cup water
¼ cup oil
  Parsley

Combine dry ingredients. Gradually stir in vinegar and water. Simmer for 8 minutes, stirring frequently. Beat oil slowly into mixture. Add parsley when serving. This dressing is delicious over greens. It is also excellent as a spread over hamburgers when ingredients such as mustard, ketchup, mayonnaise, and onions are not allowed in the diet.

What are some easy-to-follow nonallergenic dessert recipes suitable for the whole family?

Food allergy does not necessarily mean no more sweets. Rest assured—a good many allergen-free tasty desserts can be easily prepared that will please the entire family.

The following recipes will give you an idea of the many possibilities available.*

Crinkle Cups*
(egg-free, gluten-free, milk-free, wheat-free)

6 squares semisweet chocolate   2 tablespoons milk-free margarine

Heat chocolate and milk-free margarine over hot water until chocolate is partially melted. Remove from hot water and stir rapidly until ingredients are well blended and mixture is thick. Using a teaspoon, cover the inside surface of 10 large paper baking cups with a thin layer of mixture. Set in muffin pans; chill until hard. Fill with ice cream or pudding. Chill in refrigerator before peeling off paper.

Cinnamon Munch*
(egg-free, gluten-free, milk-free, wheat-free)

¼ cup sugar
1 teaspoon cinnamon
3 tablespoons milk-free margarine

3 cups Rice Chex or Corn Chex cereal

Mix sugar and cinnamon and set aside. Melt margarine in a frying pan over low heat and add cereal, stirring gently until each piece is coated. Sprinkle half the cinnamon-sugar mixture evenly over cereal, stirring to coat each piece. Continue heating, stirring, and sprinkling until all pieces are covered. Spread to cool before serving.

Ice Cream Cones*
(egg-free, gluten-free, milk-free, wheat-free)

5 cups Puffed Rice cereal
⅓ cup milk-free margarine
½ cup peanut butter

½ pound miniature marshmallows (or 32 large marshmallows)

Heat Puffed Rice cereal in shallow pan for 10 minutes in 350° F oven. Pour into large greased bowl. Melt milk-free margarine, peanut butter, and marshmallows in double boiler. Pour marshmallow mixture over Puffed Rice until mixture is coated. Pack mixture in bottom and on sides of paper cups or greased custard cups, leaving the center hollow. Chill thoroughly. Fill with ice cream when needed. (Peanut butter may be omitted.)

* Recipes marked with an asterisk (*) are courtesy of the Allergy Information Association, Weston, Ontario, Canada.

Spritz**
(wheat-free, milk-free, egg-free, corn-free)

1 cup milk-free margarine	1 teaspoon vanilla
½ cup brown sugar, packed	2⅔ cups barley flour
1 teaspoon egg substitute, plus 2 tablespoons water	6 teaspoons baking powder

(For gluten-free diets, use a cereal-free baking powder; instead of barley flour, use 2½ cups less 1⅔ tablespoons rice flour.)

Cream together the milk-free margarine and brown sugar. Beat in egg substitute, water, and vanilla. Mix together the flour and baking powder and gradually add to the creamed mixture. Mix until smooth. Force dough through cookie press onto ungreased cookie sheet. Bake in 400° F oven for 8 minutes. Makes 60 cookies.

Orient Tea Bread**
(wheat-free, milk-free, egg-free, corn-free)

½ cup milk-free margarine	½ teaspoon salt
¾ cup brown sugar, packed	7½ teaspoons baking powder
1 teaspoon egg substitute, plus 2 tablespoons water	1 teaspoon baking soda
2 teaspoons grated lemon peel	¼ teaspoon cinnamon
2 teaspoons grated orange peel (optional)	¼ teaspoon ginger
	¾ cup orange juice
3 cups barley flour	½ cup steeped tea, cooled (try jasmine or Earl Grey)

(For gluten-free diets, use a cereal-free baking powder and, for the barley flour, substitute 2⅔ cups less 1 tablespoon rice flour.)

Cream the margarine with the sugar and then add egg substitute, water, and the lemon and orange peel. Mix the barley flour with the salt, baking powder, baking soda, and spices. Add the dry ingredients to the creamed mixture alternately with the orange juice and then the tea. Bake in a greased and floured (with barley flour) 9-cup mold for 35 to 45 minutes in a 350° F oven. Cool in the pan for 10 minutes and turn onto a wire rack to continue cooling. (Variation: for tea muffins, pour batter into paper muffin cups and bake for 15 minutes.)

Cranberry Kuchen**
(wheat-free, milk-free, egg-free, corn-free)

1 teaspoon egg substitute, plus
  2 tablespoons water
½ cup sugar
½ cup water
2 tablespoons salad oil
1 cup barley flour
4 teaspoons baking powder

½ teaspoon salt
2 cups coarsely chopped fresh
  cranberries
TOPPING
¾ cup barley flour
½ cup sugar
3 tablespoons milk-free margarine

(For gluten-free diets, use a cereal-free baking powder and, for the barley flour, substitute 1 cup rice flour less 2 tablespoons; for the topping, substitute 1 cup rice flour less 1½ tablespoons.)

Beat the egg substitute with the 2 tablespoons of water; then combine with sugar, water, and salad oil. Mix together the flour, baking powder, salt. Stir and add to sugar mixture. Blend well. Pour batter into a greased 8-inch square pan. Sprinkle top with cranberries. For topping, combine the flour and sugar and cut in the milk-free margarine. Bake at 375° F for 25 to 30 minutes. Delicious when served warm.

Banana Supreme Cake**
(wheat-free, milk-free, egg-free, corn-free)

1¼ cups sugar
½ cup shortening
2 teaspoons egg substitute, plus
  4 tablespoons water
1 tablespoon fresh lemon juice
2 medium bananas, mashed

1½ cups barley flour
½ teaspoon mace (optional)
3¾ teaspoons baking powder
1 teaspoon baking soda
¼ cup water

(For gluten-free diets, use a cereal-free baking powder and, for the barley flour, substitute 1⅓ cups rice flour less 2 tablespoons.)

Cream together the sugar and shortening. Add the egg substitute and water and lemon juice and beat well. Mix in the mashed bananas. Stir together the flour, mace, baking powder, and baking soda. Add the flour mixture and the ¼ cup water alternately to the creamed mixture, beginning and ending with flour. Grease and flour (with barley flour) a 9-cup mini-Bundt pan. Bake in a 350° F oven for 40 minutes. Cool in pan for 15 minutes. Remove from pan and complete cooling on a wire rack.

Jelly Bellies**
(wheat-free, milk-free, egg-free, corn-free)

½ cup brown sugar	2½ cups barley flour
½ cup milk-free margarine	6 teaspoons baking powder
1 teaspoon almond flavoring	½ teaspoon salt
2 teaspoons egg substitute, plus	
4 tablespoons water	

(For gluten-free diets, use a cereal-free baking powder and substitute for barley flour, 2¼ cups rice flour less 1 tablespoon.)

Cream together sugar and milk-free margarine. Beat in remaining ingredients. Chill briefly. Roll into 1-inch balls and roll balls in sugar. Place on lightly greased and floured (with barley flour) sheet. Bake for 5 minutes in 375° F oven. Remove from oven and make a thumbprint in each cookie. Continue baking for about 8 more minutes. When cool, fill each thumbprint with a dab of jelly. Makes 42 cookies.

What kind of nonallergenic food products are available and where can they be found?

Below is a selected list of companies that manufacture food products for restricted diets, including diets prescribed by doctors for allergic patients. (Check with your doctor first, however, to determine if these products are suitable for your or your child's particular, special diet.)

When searching for a particular product, call up your local supermarket to see if it is in stock. If that store does not have the product you want, the store manager may be able to refer you to another supermarket or grocery store in the area that does.

Are there any associations and/or agencies that can help answer questions related to food allergy?

The following government agencies and nonprofit associations can help you with questions on food composition, food product labels, and food additives:

American Allergy Association
P. O. Box 7273
Menlo Park, CA 94025

Allergy Information Association
25 Poynter Dr., Room 7
Weston, Ontario M9R 1K8 Canada

American Dietetic Association
430 North Michigan Ave.
Chicago, IL 60611

Consumer Communications
Room 15 B-32
U.S. Food and Drug Administration
5600 Fishers Lane
Rockville, MD 20852

Human Nutrition Center
U.S. Department of Agriculture
Fourteenth St. and Independence Ave. SW
Washington, DC 20850

Much of the material in this chapter is based on information provided by the Allergy Information Association.

Table 8.4. Manufacturers of Products for Restricted Diets

COMPANY	PRODUCTS	AVAILABILITY
Chicago Dietetic Supply 405 E. Shawmut Ave. LaGrange, IL 60525 (312) 352-6900	Wheat-, corn-, and gluten-free: Featherweight brand (formerly Cellu) flours and starches Cereal-free: Featherweight baking powder Corn-free: Juice-packed and water-packed canned fruit (no corn syrup)	Supermarkets, health food stores, mail order (food sent via UPS)
El Molino Mills P.O. Box 2156 345 N. Baldwin Park Blvd. City of Industry, CA 91746 (213) 962-7167	Chocolate-free: Caracoa confections, cookies, and candy bars (made with carob) Wheat-free: Cookies (made with barley flour)	Supermarkets, health food stores, candy counters
Ener-G-Foods 6901 Fox Ave. S. Seattle, WA 98124	Wheat-free: Ener-G-Foods rice bread; potato, rice, corn, barley, and oat mix (flour replacements); pizza; cookies Egg-free: Ener-G-Foods Egg Replacer (formerly Jolly Joan) powdered egg replacement Gluten- and lactose-free: Soyquik (for baking and drinking)	Mixes: Health food stores Baked goods: Mail order (food sent via UPS)
Fearn Soya Foods 1206 N. 31st St. Melrose Park, IL 60160 (312) 345-2335	Gluten-free: Fearn Soya or Naturfresh brand rice baking mix, rice flour, nonfat dry milk, soya granules, natural soya powder, Qualipro Shake Mix (carob, chocolate, and vanilla flavors) Milk-free: Bran muffin mix, cornbread mix, pancake mix	Natural and health food stores, mail order (full cases only)

Manufacturers of Products for Restricted Diets (cont.)

COMPANY	PRODUCTS	AVAILABILITY
General Mills, Inc. 9200 Wayzata Blvd. Minneapolis, MN 55440 (612) 540-2311	Corn-free: granola bars, granola cereals, Cheerios cereal, Wheathearts Cereal Write for lists of chocolate-free, wheat-free, milk-free, and egg-free products	Supermarkets
Gerber Baby Foods, Inc. 445 S. State St. Fremont, MI 49412 (616) 928-2000	Milk-free: Meat-Base Formula (MBF) (for infants) Write for list of gluten-free, corn-free, wheat-free, citrus-free, egg-free, and milk-free baby foods	Supermarkets
Hain Pure Food Co., Inc. 13660 S. Figueroa Los Angeles, CA 90061 (213) 538-9922	Egg-free: Hain Eggless Imitation Mayonnaise Corn-free: Hain salad dressings Milk-free: Safflower margarine	Supermarkets, health and natural food stores
Heinz U.S.A. (baby food) Consumer Relations Dept. P.O. Box 57 Pittsburgh, PA 15230 (412) 237-5757	Milk-, wheat-, egg-, and citrus-free: Oatmeal cereal with apples and bananas, rice cereal with apples and bananas Gluten-, milk-, egg-, wheat-, and citrus-free: Apples and pears, applesauce, apple and apricots; all fruit juices except orange juice and Orange-Apple-Banana Juice Drink which both contain citrus Write for their booklet, "Planning Meals for the Allergic Infant"	Supermarkets

Manufacturers of Products for Restricted Diets (cont.)

COMPANY	PRODUCTS	AVAILABILITY
Henkel Corp. Special Dietary Dept. 4620 West 77th Minneapolis, MN 55435 (612) 830-7831	Wheat-free: Aproten paste products (cornstarch-based)	Supermarkets, health food stores, mail order
Loma Linda Foods 11503 Pierce Riverside, CA 92505 (714) 785-2444	Milk-free: Soyagen (for adults); Soyalac (for infants) Milk-free and corn-free: I-Soyalac (for infants) Wheat-free: Nutina (vegetable protein loaf), Vitaburger Yeast-free: Nutina	Supermarkets (in California), health food stores
Ralston-Purina Co. Checkerboard Square St. Louis, MO 63188 (314) 982-1000	Wheat-free: Corn Chex, Rice Chex, Rykrisp	Supermarkets
Rich Products Corp. 1149 Niagara Buffalo, NY 14213 (716) 878-8000	Milk-free: Coffee Rich (liquid nondairy creamer), Richwhip (whipped topping in liquid form), Rich's Whip Topping (aerosol form)	Supermarkets, in frozen foods section
Vita-Wheat Baked Products, Inc. 1839 Hilton Rd. Ferndale, MI 48220 (313) 543-0888	Wheat-, egg-, and milk-free: Rice bread (also corn-free); rice flour; soybean flour (contains potato starch); apple, apricot butter, and carob cookies (contain potato starch); sandwich bread (contains yeast and oil) Wheat-free and citrus-free: Fruit cake (contains potato starch)	Health food stores, mail order (food sent via UPS)

CHAPTER 9

All about Asthma
by Sheldon L. Spector, M.D.

Not all the material in this chapter applies uniformly to every patient. Only by working closely with your physician can you understand your condition and improve it.

Definition, Significance, and Incidence

Although asthma is a common disorder, it is difficult to define accurately, even for a physician. Using data from many sources, physicians know that the incidence of this condition is relatively high. Asthma affects nearly nine million people in the United States and causes an estimated four thousand deaths each year. It may also be an underlying cause of death in three to four times that number. Moreover, it isn't evident from these figures that asthma causes considerable discomfort and inconvenience. Asthma may keep as many as thirty thousand working people from their jobs each day, not to mention the students kept home from school. Asthmatics frequently wind up in emergency rooms because of this disease or its complications.

To the patient, asthma is a feeling of tightness in the chest, labored breathing, wheezing, coughing, gasping, and fatigue, with the apprehension that results. Although not all these symptoms may be present during a specific attack, the patient is always acutely aware that something uncomfortable and unpleasant is going on in his or her body.

To the physician, asthma is a reversible, obstructive disease of the air passages that is caused by varying degrees of bronchial muscle spasm, a swelling of the mucosa, and an excessive amount of mucus. The bronchial muscles of an asthmatic twitch more than do the muscles of a normal person. This is evident in the bronchial obstruction that occurs after inhalation of small quantities of histamine, for example, or of another chemical substance that resembles acteylcholine, a substance normally released from certain nerve endings. Five points about the definition of asthma should be understood:

1. The term *reversible* is important to the patient. It means that, with the appropriate medication, the patient's breathing condition will improve and eventually become normal. It is an optimistic outlook, since the physician need only find the right approach or combination of approaches and the patient can return to a relatively normal life. If lung damage has occurred, however, some effects of asthma may be irreversible. In such cases, patients will never be able to breathe as well as they once could. If this happens, the aim in treating asthmatics is to help them function as well as possible under the circumstances. It is sometimes difficult, however, to determine the extent to which a patient's disease is reversible. Only after trying bronchodilators, and even long-term corticosteroids, can we properly assess the prospect of reversibility.

2. "Wheezing"—in the popular mind the most common symptom of asthma—is more often than not the doctor's term, not the patient's. Patients usually mention a feeling of tightness during an asthma attack. Coughing is another symptom that may occur, either alone in an individual not suspecting a diagnosis of asthma, or as part of an asthma attack. Some patients also experience a feeling of fatigue during an attack.

3. Many people, including some physicians, confuse asthma with allergy. Numerous asthma patients, in fact, do not have allergies, and many allergy patients do not have asthma. Perhaps this confusion has led patients to seek a magic cure for asthma by eliminating some allergic substance in the environment. Unfortunately, because asthma is a complex condition with many causes, people are rarely able to remove a single environmental substance and thus significantly alter their condition. Realistically, they should not expect a cure but rather seek a program of treatment adequate for controlling the symptoms of wheezing and one that will allow them to live fairly normal lives.

4. Some of the same misconceptions discussed in paragraph 3 have led to an incorrect or oversimplified definition of asthma, primarily because of the use of the adjectives *extrinsic* and *intrinsic*. These are outmoded terms that no longer indicate accurately the outcome of treatment. The term *extrinsic asthma* refers to people in whom allergies seem to be the most important causative factors. Skin tests are usually positive. The patient is often a child or young adult rather than someone who has developed asthma later in life.

Such asthma attacks are thought to be related to such specific allergens as ragweed. Doctors now doubt that such a pure group exists, since such factors as irritants and emotions may play as large a role in this allergic group as any other subgroup. It is rare for just a few environmental substances to be responsible for all the symptoms. That situation exists only among the mildest asthmatic patients, those that respond readily to treatment. At present, the term *intrinsic asthma* is used to refer to patients who are not allergic, whose asthma attacks do not stem from a known cause but are triggered by infection and nonspecific irritants. The word *intrinsic*, however, does not describe accurately a specific, known mechanism. This situation arises—in the case of bacteria, at least—because of the role of infection in provoking symptoms in asthmatic patients, a role that is uncertain. When these terms fit a patient's condition very well, the word *mixed* is used. A "mixed asthmatic" patient is one whose symptoms are triggered by extrinsic factors and who has persistent problems with unknown causes.

5. What the allergist calls an intrinsic asthmatic, a chest physician might call chronic bronchitis. *Chronic bronchitis* is defined as a condition in which a cough with sputum is present for at least three months of the year and for at least two consecutive years. Many physicians, however, are not satisfied with this term. The amount of sputum can vary in an individual, and medications can greatly decrease the amount of sputum. Many "bronchitics" have irritable airways similar to those of asthmatic patients. Because reversibility is almost always present, treatment of these patients is usually no different from that of other asthmatics. Perhaps where bronchitics differ most is that many of them have a long history of smoking and thus less chance of reversibility.

What Causes Asthma?

The actual cause, or causes, of asthma is not known. To develop asthma, it is probably necessary for a person to be predisposed genetically, and to be exposed to such environmental factors as infections or to allergens such as house dust and mold.

Some people develop a condition similar to asthma after a viral infection. When the infection clears, the patient's airways continue to be irritated. Thus one important difference between an asthmatic and a person in normal health is the persistence of bronchial obstruction after an infection. The viral theory, then, is one possible explanation for the development of asthma. From a practical point of view, although the physician does not necessarily know the cause of the asthma, he or she can prescribe treatment that takes into account many of the causative factors.

The human body must constantly try to overcome those forces that would lead to continuous bronchial obstruction. Its success is obvious, since the asthmatic does not wheeze or experience tightness all of the time. Asthma is characterized by periods of ups and downs. It is also true that relatively mild bronchial obstruction which may not be apparent to the patient will show up in breathing tests in a doctor's office. If many stimuli are responsible for a given amount of broncho-constriction in a patient, the elimination of one or more stimuli might result in sufficient improvement for the patient to be aware of the improvement.

A patient may mistakenly perceive a cause-and-effect relationship between an environmental stimulus and the bronchial obstruction that seems to result from it. Many stimuli are more important in causing an attack when the patient is about to wheeze than when the patient is relatively symptom-free. Misunderstanding of this relationship has led to some current myths about asthma. One example, is the woman who develops asthma at the time of her husband's death. She forgets how run-down she was and about the infection she acquired earlier. Her asthma might inappropriately be called psychogenic. Another example is the man who develops asthma during the Christmas season and who is convinced that the Christmas tree was the cause. He overlooks the upper respiratory infection and other problems that occurred simultaneously. Still another example is the man who ascribes his asthma to his mother-in-law. He develops symptoms in her house but overlooks the possibility that her cat is responsible.

The physician familiar with the body mechanisms that provoke wheezing is in the best position to help the patient understand these mechanisms. The patient should also keep in mind that asthma itself is not a simple illness, that approaches used by different physicians may vary. The interested reader should note the following points.

1. Patients differ with respect to the causes of attacks. In some cases, infections seem to play a major role; in others, stimulants such as strong odors, exercise, laughing, or cold air are important. In still other patients, a truly allergic reaction may be the most important factor.

2. Patients differ with respect to the location of the major areas of obstruction. Some seem to have obstruction primarily in their

large breathing tubes, whereas others have it mainly in their small breathing tubes; others have obstruction in both. The collapsibility of bronchial tubes also varies, and this can affect breathing tests. Some patients trap too much air and thus overexpand their lungs.

3. Patients differ in how much the obstruction in their airways can be reversed. The concept of reversibility has already been mentioned. The most common test of reversibility is the patient's reaction to an aerosolized bronchodilator such as Isuprel Mistometer or Bronkosol. Some people require prolonged, around-the-clock therapy, which often includes daily or every-other-day steroid therapy before normal breathing is regained. Despite much medication, many improve their bronchial airway obstruction but never return to a normal state. Patients with obstructive airways disease who show no evidence of reversibility even after the most rigorous therapy program known may suffer from a serious condition such as emphysema. These patients, however, do not have asthma.

4. People differ in their response to various medications. Some are "responders" to many of the medications used in the treatment of asthma, and some are "nonresponders."

5. People also differ as to the amount of medication necessary to produce the desired effect. It may take eight times longer for one person to eliminate theophylline (the most common antiasthmatic medication) from the body than it does for another. Thus the dose necessary for controlling asthma symptoms may vary significantly from one person to another.

Indications of Asthma

A patient who is examined between attacks may appear normal. Usually, though, wheezing caused by forced expiration is detectable in the chest. During a severe attack, the patient may use both belly and neck muscles to breathe. The chest may expand, the person may turn blue and lose fluid through sweating, and the heart may begin to beat rapidly (although this is sometimes caused by the medication used to treat asthma attacks). The absence of wheezing during a severe attack could actually be a bad sign, indicating that the bronchial tubes have filled with mucus.

In the next few pages we discuss some factors that contribute to the onset of asthma.

Hereditary

Although genetic factors are important, they should not be over-emphasized. The absence of a family history of allergy does not mean that someone cannot have an allergy. By the same token, a family history of allergy does not mean that the patient cannot have a non-allergic cause for his asthma. People inherit at least two important components that do not necessarily come from the same genes: the immunologic responses involving antibodies responsible for an allergic reaction, and organ hyperreactivity, or "twitchy lung." Inheritance becomes even more complicated when other possible genetic factors are considered, such as the number and location of the cells that release asthma-triggering substances. Even the blood supply to these cells is suspect.

Immunologic

The immune system of the human body is extremely complex. Four types of immune reactions have been studied and described, two of which may be responsible for some common allergic problems. When a foreign substance enters the body, the body's response is to manufacture a defensive substance called an antibody. The antibody has a shape similar to that of the foreign substance; this enables the antibody to attach itself to the substance, much as two pieces of a jigsaw puzzle fit together, and deactivate it. Some antibodies are protective, while others contribute to adverse reactions such as sneezing and wheezing. The antibody known as immunoglobulin E is associated with most immediate allergic reactions, for example, those associated with hay fever and asthma. A Type I reaction occurs when an allergic foreign substance combines with immunoglobulin E. Wheezing may also accompany the interaction between a foreign substance such as mold and immunoglobulin G (which is usually protective). This type of antibody causes a Type III reaction. Immunologic processes that work through certain blood cells of the body, causing a Type IV reaction, may contribute to the reactions mentioned above; but just how this type of interaction works has not yet been determined. As knowledge of these immunologic reactions increases, physicians will be better able to characterize allergic diseases and treat them.

Physiological

Tests of breathing are called pulmonary function tests. They measure the capacity of the lungs to stretch, the volume of air that flows through them, the extent of obstruction to airflow, and the distribution of air in the chest. Tests can be administered that compare the supply of blood with the supply of air in the lungs, and measure a patient's response to various medications so that the patient can be given the most effective medication.

In attempting to diagnose reversible lung disease, several types of bronchodilators, and even corticosteroids, may have to be tried. If the patient still does not respond, a diagnosis of irreversible lung disease is reached.

Psychological

Over a period of a few years, some hospitalized asthmatic patients were asked to fill out a questionnaire listing the symptoms they experienced during an asthma attack. Seventy-seven symptoms were recorded and divided into five symptom categories. Patients experiencing much panic and fear during an asthma attack needed to be on high doses of the most potent medications. They also requested more medication from their doctors even though their pulmonary function tests revealed little change. This high panic-fever response may actually contribute to patients' personal view of themselves as invalids, and therefore as being more vulnerable to an asthma attack. Such patients may also overmedicate, thus becoming more susceptible to side effects that could otherwise be avoided. On the other hand, patients with a low panic-fear response requested medication infrequently even when they needed treatment.

Like other groups of patients with chronic illnesses, asthmatic patients develop various ways of coping with their asthma. When they believe they must yield to the disease, they often do so, with the result that they make their condition worse. This is often true of children who find that they get more attention from their parents and families when they are ill.

Some patients respond to suggestion; others do not. A suggestible patient might experience tightness in the chest just at the thought of contact with a cat or a dog. Even an artificial rose can induce tightness if the stimulus is a reminder of a previous bronchoconstriction. By identifying this group of asthma patients, physicians can prescribe treatment programs that minimize the power of suggestion during an asthma attack.

Biochemical

Biochemical factors are difficult to understand, and new theories are constantly being proposed. The body contains specialized cells that have attachment sites on their surface with which chemicals interact. These sites, called receptors, are divided into three main groups: alpha adrenergic, beta adrenergic, and cholinergic. The interaction of these receptors corresponds to changes in cyclic adenosine monophosphate (cyclic AMP). Formation of cyclic AMP causes a favorable response, since the formation is related to bronchodilation and prevention of the release of chemicals within the cells involved in bronchoconstriction. Another substance—cyclic guanosine monophosphate (cyclic GMP)—is thought to have the opposite effect: *contributing* to bronchoconstriction. The influence of the cholinergic receptor is exerted through cyclic GMP. Researchers and physicians believe that cigarette smoke, automobile fumes, and strong odors contribute to the interaction of these substances.

The medications commonly used in treating asthma are thought to work through cyclic AMP and cyclic GMP biochemical pathways. Epinephrine, isoproterenol, metaproterenol, and terbutaline stimulate cyclic AMP formation and cause bronchodilation. Theophylline inhibits cyclic AMP breakdown, producing the same net effect. Phenotolamine sometimes causes bronchodilation by increasing cyclic AMP. Through another mechanism, such substances as atropine block cyclic GMP levels and produce bronchodilation. Corticosteroids seem to affect beta adrenergic receptors as one of their modes of action. A recent theory of asthma suggests that an antibody is directed against the beta adrenergic receptor.

Hormonal

Although hormonal factors are probably important, data explaining their exact role are insufficient. Among some women, asthmatic symptoms have been found to worsen during menstrual periods or during pregnancy. Other patients may develop a severe worsening of their asthma, along with a hyperactive thyroid; improvement is possible only after the thyroid condition is treated.

Clinical

Although, historically, the most common complaint of the asthmatic patient is tightness in the chest, other common symptoms of asthma are cough, wheezing, and shortness of breath, followed by symptom-free periods. Among some people, a persistent chronic cough, especially at night, or shortness of breath, with a heavy production of sputum, are the main symptoms. Wheezing is a sound made by a rapid flow of air through the airways. As is true of a musical instrument, sound is produced only when the airflow is sufficient. The lungs of some patients may be too tight for them to wheeze; in these people, mucus plugs block the flow of air through the bronchial tubes. An asthmatic usually has hyperinflated lungs, which means air is trapped and cannot be expelled during normal expiration. When the lung is in this expanded condition, the patient must work harder to breathe and thus tires more easily.

Diagnosis of Asthma

A diagnosis of asthma is indicated when a patient has a history of wheezing after exposure to specific environmental substances or respiratory infections and is suffering from generalized obstruction of the air passages.

Although many physicians place great emphasis on family histories, these histories are not invariably important. Lack of history neither proves nor disproves that the patient has asthma. On the other hand, a previous history of eczema, hay fever, nasal polyps, or sinusitis should alert the physician to the possibility of asthma.

Chest X-Rays and EKGs

A chest x-ray may appear either normal or overinflated, with the diaphragm pushed down. An electrocardiogram (EKG) is usually normal. During a severe attack, right-sided heart strain or enlargement may occur.

Skin Tests

Skin tests are used to distinguish a group of asthmatics who have allergies. Such tests alone, however, do not make possible a diagnosis of asthma.

Bronchial Inhalation Challenge

Bronchial inhalation challenges with antigens might also help define an immunoglobulin-mediated cause for the asthma. A positive bronchial inhalation challenge to methacholine (a substance similar to acetylcholine) or histamine may help confirm a diagnosis that is unclear, such as might result in a patient with only a chronic cough.

Studies of Sputum and Blood

Eosinophils are certain types of blood cells often associated with asthma. Their presence in relatively large amounts in the blood, sputum, or nasal secretions is frequently seen in symptomatic allergic states.

Pulmonary Function Tests

Pulmonary function tests are helpful as indicators of the severity of the asthma, the degree of reversibility, and the likely response to certain treatments.

Measuring Arterial Blood Gases

Arterial blood gases are measured to evaluate the severity of the asthma. The blood is usually low in oxygen during a severe attack. At first, the patient may be breathing so fast that more carbon dioxide than usual is breathed out. A patient who becomes fatigued will retain carbon dioxide and thus risk respiratory failure.

Variant Diagnoses of Asthma

Almost anything that causes narrowing or obstruction of the bronchial tree may be associated with wheezing and similar symptoms. Foreign matter, trauma, pneumonia, and tumors can produce such narrowing. Some forms of heart disease resemble asthma, and cardiac failure is sometimes diagnosed as wheezing. Blood clots that move from the legs to the lungs, and tumors that produce chemical substances, can also provoke wheezing. Poisoning by insecticides or other cholinergic drugs can induce bronchoconstriction. Certain environmental exposures can bring on asthmalike symptoms, while other diseases such as Löffler's syndrome and polyarteritis nodosa sometimes resemble asthma. In some foreign countries, parasitic infestation of the lungs must also be considered a possibility among people apparently suffering from asthma. Finally, the upper airway obstruction sometimes found after a tracheotomy can cause wheezing that is audible throughout the lungs.

The two most common pulmonary problems that are confused with asthma are chronic bronchitis and emphysema. Although the mechanisms involved in these diseases appear to differ, the symptoms are remarkably similar. Chronic bronchitis is an inflammation of the

bronchial airways resulting in coughing and excessive mucous secretion. Bronchospasm may also be a major factor, in which case treatment would be similar to that of chronic asthma. Many patients with
chronic bronchitis later develop emphysema. A sustained, low level
of oxygen in the blood, along with cardiac problems, is more characteristic of a patient with chronic bronchitis than of a patient suffering
from asthma.

Diagnosis of emphysema, another disease commonly confused with
asthma, should be applied to a destructive process in the lungs involving the air sacs and air ducts. Air sacs that are unaffected often
compensate, becoming larger and larger and resulting in a decrease
in the blood surface exposed to the gas in extended air sacs. The result of this process is a diminished capacity for the exchange of oxygen and carbon dioxide, accompanied by a loss of elasticity in the
tissue, so that the patient cannot inflate and empty the lungs spontaneously. The lungs of an emphysema patient seem to remain in-
flated. Because emphysema rarely exists in isolation, asthma is
sometimes mistaken for emphysema. In either case, the reversible
symptoms are all that can be treated.

Treating a Severe Attack of Asthma

The best time to treat a severe attack of asthma is several days before it happens. Complications such as infection or exposure to allergens may be responsible. At the same time, the fault may lie with the
patient, the physician, or both. Occasionally a patient visits the emergency room, receives treatment in the form of epinephrine (Adrenalin), and improves enough to be sent home—only to return with
severe problems later that day or the next. Such a course of treatment
contributes to the development of a severe asthma attack.

In discussing the treatment of a severe attack of asthma, I am as-
suming that a diagnosis of asthma has already been made, and that
the physician is aware that other problems may be present. Certain
complications of severe asthma, such as seepage of air from the lungs
into the chest cavity, must also be ruled out. Once laboratory tests
have been performed, a diagnosis is made and a treatment program is
selected, based on the seriousness of the patient's case:

Hospitalization. A hospital is the best environment in which to
treat severe cases of asthma. The ideal environment is a respiratory
intensive care unit operated by specialists and equipped with con-

tinuous monitoring equipment. Repetitive blood-gas tests (which measure the levels of oxygen and carbon dioxide, as well as acid-base relationships) are necessary for the physician to decide whether breathing assistance is needed. Whether oxygen and sodium bicarbonate are used depends on the patient's clinical condition.

Intravenous fluids. Fluids are given intravenously to help thin out mucous secretions and to provide a blood line (a route kept open for the quick delivery of fluids and medications) for the intravenous administration of medication. A considerable amount of fluid (at least two and one-half quarts) should be given to an adult unless there are indications that this is unsafe.

Aminophylline. Aminophylline is administered intravenously to ensure that the dose reaches the appropriate blood levels.

Aerosolized bronchodilator. An aerosolized bronchodilator such as isoetharine (Bronkosol) or metaproterenol (Alupent or Metaprel) can be used fairly often if the patient has not previously overused them.

Intravenous corticosteroids. Although physicians do not fully understand the function of corticosteroids, they do know that intravenous corticosteroids enhance the effect of certain bronchodilators.

Epinephrine or terbutaline sulfate. Given by injection, epinephrine or terbutaline are helpful, especially in treating young children. These drugs may have to be avoided, or at least used cautiously, by older people susceptible to cardiac problems. Intravenous therapy has the advantage of better controlling the administration of bronchodilators and ensuring that enough fluid is present to remove liquid secretions. After the mucus plugs are loosened, postural drainage becomes more effective. A common mistake is to stop intravenous therapy prematurely. The patient often urges the physician to discontinue this therapy, but the physician should not do so until certain that the maximum benefit has been achieved. Only at this time should oral therapy be instituted.

Managing Chronic Symptoms in Asthmatic Patients

Because asthma is a chronic illness, it becomes a source of frustration to everyone involved. It is frustrating to patients who would like to deny its existence, as well as to families which must devote considerable time and money to treatment. It is frustrating to busy hospital physicians, who must see patients in emergency rooms even when they know patients have already responded to treatment with epinephrine. And it is frustrating to private physicians, who receive repeated calls at night from asthmatic patients in trouble. Eventually, some physicians become convinced that patients' asthma is imaginary.

A chronic illness such as asthma must be treated appropriately through frequent follow-up visits. The physician must listen to the patient for clues to the patient's condition, then try to determine whether the condition has an organic origin or is merely "in the patient's head." Patients must also be taught to recognize variations in their symptoms and to seek medical help as early as possible when these symptoms occur. The patient must share much of the responsibility for treatment, with the physician serving as a guide.

Avoiding Asthma Attacks

The task of continuously avoiding stimulants—for example, airborne pollens and nonspecific irritants such as car exhaust and perfumes, which pervade the environment—is often difficult if not impossible. People who live or work in areas where these stimulants are concentrated should (or must) wear special masks. A smoke-filled room may not only be uncomfortable for an asthmatic, but the smoke can actually provoke an attack. People suffering from asthma should unquestionably not smoke; smoking can lead to a worse condition or to the development of chronic bronchitis or emphysema.

Although contributing factors such as changes in barometric pressure, temperature, or humidity are often impossible to regulate, an individual *can* avoid sitting in front of fans or air conditioners. If this person goes out in the cold air, the mouth and nose should be covered with a scarf or a special mask should be worn. Although allergic reactions to potent food allergens such as nuts and seafood are not common in adults, these reactions do occur, and suspect foods should be avoided. Because it is difficult for children to keep away from certain foods, their parents should be all the more attentive. Food allergies are best diagnosed by using an elimination diet or a double-blind ingestion technique. Severe elimination diets, especially those embarked upon by the patient without a physician's guidance, can eventually lead to malnutrition or even near starvation.

The patient who knows he or she is allergic should try to remove irritating factors from the environment. For example, a room should not be dusted by someone allergic to house dust, nor should that person mow the lawn if grass is an irritant.

The hazards that exist in work environments, to which people are exposed over fairly long periods, have been recognized for centuries. The potentially harmful effect of hazardous substances, and the treatment required, are, however, beyond the scope of this chapter.

Aspirin and compounds containing aspirin and other pain relievers can cause adverse reactions and even death in some asthmatic patients. A large number of people develop bronchial obstruction from tartrazine (FD and C#5), a common yellow coloring found in foods ranging from margarine to hot dogs and in many yellow or orange medications. Aspirin is easily avoided; there are reasonably safe substitutes such as acetaminophen (Tylenol). To avoid an adverse reaction to tartrazine, a special test called a double-blind oral challenge should be performed. This test requires the taking, on different days, of capsules that appear to be identical. One capsule contains the active drug, whereas the other contains an inert substance such as sugar. Neither the physician nor the patient knows what the pill contains at the time of the test, hence the term *double-blind*.

Alcoholic beverages may adversely affect some asthmatic patients. Although exactly how this occurs is not always clear, the reaction can be triggered by an ingredient such as yeast or by the effect of alcohol on cell tissues. Moreover, alcohol can interact as a drug with other medications taken by other patients.

Avoiding emotional tension is always a good general rule to follow, and techniques are available for relaxing the air passages.

Self-Care

Sinus, Nasal, and Bronchial Disease

In my experience, about 60 percent of asthma patients have sinus disease that can be detected by x-rays. In many cases, sinus disease goes unrecognized because clinical symptoms may be minor or absent. Sinus infection can spread to the breathing tubes and lungs. It is important to clear a site of any infection that can spread to the lower respiratory tract. Chronic nasal drip is another common problem of asthmatic patients. It is often associated with a drip down the back of the throat. A simple salt solution administered two or three times a day can prevent secretions from accumulating in the lower respiratory tract. This solution can be purchased in a drugstore or prepared by the patient. It is poured into the cupped hand and sniffed or, if purchased, administered by following the manufacturer's directions.

Certain postural drainage techniques can be learned and used to drain mucus. These techniques are often used, along with certain liquids and bronchodilator medications, especially when mucus plugs and/or secretions are a problem. Patients with bronchitis have found postural drainage techniques particularly useful. They can even be administered by a spouse, friend, or relative. These techniques involve positioning the patient properly, to promote drainage, and gently clapping on the patient's chest with cupped hands. Postural drainage positions are designed to increase the drainage of mucus from all areas of the lungs. The idea is to place the affected area of the chest uppermost so that gravity can assist drainage. Occasionally, however, when the bronchospasm is not adequately controlled, a patient's condition worsens with this approach. This treatment should be used only with certain patients and at selected times, often accompanied by an aerosolized bronchodilator and following a physician's instructions.

Breathing Techniques

Breathing techniques taught by a physical therapist or a physician may prove useful in stopping or at least relieving an asthma attack. Breathing becomes even more important during periods of stress or increased activity; it should be done through the nose, slowly and smoothly, and the air should be released slowly from the lungs. The upper chest should be relaxed, and an attempt should be made to fill the lower part of the lungs. The entire chest and abdomen move when a person breathes deeply. Changes of position may also help, for example, lying down, sitting, leaning forward while sitting on a pillow, and sitting and leaning forward with a straight back.

Obesity

An overweight patient must breathe more and pump more blood to supply extra food to cells. All this requires energy. Because corticosteroids can increase the appetite, asthmatics should be advised that such medication can lead to weight gain. Working together, a concerned doctor and an informed patient can limit uncontrolled weight gain and thus greatly reduce this avoidable complication.

Physical Fitness

Proper exercise will not only help a patient lose weight, it will also help maintain better health and functioning of the body. By exercising, a person gradually increases his or her capacity, as well as lowering the heart rate for a given exercise. This increased capacity is what is known popularly as keeping fit. For asthmatics, however, certain exercises should be carefully monitored by a physician or a physical therapist. Medication is sometimes given just before exercise to prevent subsequent difficulty. Various medications should be tried and coordinated under the supervision of a physician.

Education

A thorough explanation of the benefits and side effects of all medication helps the patient develop a positive attitude and improves cooperation between patient and physician. Various techniques may be used, such as teaching displays of drugs commonly used, along with the primary function of each. The patient may, for example, be told the potential hazards of the medicines involved, and asked to memorize their names. Discussion groups monitored by nurses, physicians, and/or other personnel help patients understand their diseases and increase their knowledge of drug therapy.

Mental Outlook

Because we know that psychology plays an important role in physical health, techniques designed to teach patients to cope psychologically with asthma can and should be employed. These techniques may be learned in an environment specially suited to individual therapy, or they may be taught in a group-therapy environment. Either way, the therapy usually centers on the alteration of asthma-related, inappropriate behavior and adherence to a program of medication. Some patients must be taught to avoid breathing too fast (hyperventilation), since hyperventilation itself can provoke an asthma attack. Unfortunately, there are no standardized approaches to the treatment of asthmatics; therefore, individualized therapy must be employed, because of the differences in individuals and the different forms symptoms may take.

Therapeutic Agents

Theophylline Derivatives

In the United States, theophylline is the mainstay of therapy for asthma. The most common form of the drug is aminophylline, which comes in tablet, liquid, or suppository form. The oral form is usually preferred. Aminophylline suppositories should be avoided because of their erratic absorption. The breakdown and excretion of theophylline differs considerably from one patient to another; one patient may take an amount of theophylline five or ten times greater than another patient's dose. Theophylline is usually prescribed on a twenty-four-hour schedule, although longer-acting theophylline preparations are being marketed that allow a dosage rate of every eight to twelve hours. Many patients continue to take a dosage based on a six-hour schedule. The physician ascertains the patient's proper dose by obtaining a blood theophylline determination. As is true of any medication, theophylline has potential side effects; nervousness is the most common, but nausea, vomiting, and headache may also occur. These symptoms are often the first sign of too much theophylline. An overdose can even provoke convulsions. The way theophylline is metabolized—hence, its level in the blood—can change in certain circumstances, for example, when a patient has heart failure or liver disease, develops prolonged fever, smokes cigarettes, or takes certain antibiotics. Some diets can also affect theophylline metabolism. Theophylline is one of the most common ingredients in combination asthma medicines such as Tedral and Marax. Occasionally, a physician may prescribe one of these combination products, but in general it is difficult to custom-make a product, that is, proportion ingredients for a particular individual. The side effects that accompany some combination products may not be caused by theophylline but by another ingredient. Because one medication sometimes interacts with another, a particular medication can either lessen or increase the effect of the other. Caffeine (found in coffee) and theobromine (commonly found in tea) react similarly to theophylline. The doctor should know whether the patient is a heavy coffee, tea, or cola drinker, since high consumption of these beverages can increase the effect of theophylline. The patient should also tell the physician exactly what medications he or she is taking, even when the physician forgets to ask, or when there is a change in the rate of consumption or in the patient's condition. Vitamin pills and laxatives should not be forgotten, especially if the patient is taking large amounts of them. Another side effect that can occur with theophylline (or with almost any other bronchodilator medication taken orally) involves the point at which the esophagus joins the stomach. A valvelike muscle there connects the two and prevents any material in the stomach from backing up into the esophagus. Theophylline relaxes this muscle so that regurgitation of stomach contents into the esophagus occurs, resulting in a condition popularly known as heartburn. These symptoms are easily treated with an antacid to help neutralize food contents in the stomach. Other measures, such as raising the head of the bed or lying at a particular angle, sometimes help prevent this backward flow or reflux.

Aerosolized Bronchodilators

Certain medications are administered as liquids or as inhalants in canisters triggered to deliver a predetermined amount of medication. These medications often provoke fewer side effects than do similar drugs taken orally. In recent years, pharmaceutical companies have concentrated on providing drugs that selectively cause the airways to open (bronchodilation) but which do not stimulate the heart to beat faster. Another goal is to lengthen the duration of action of the drugs. Many can be diluted with sterile water or saline solution and administered with a pump (such as a Maximist) or a bulb nebulizer. Although positive pressure ventilators such as IPPB machines are another way of delivering a medication, they have not proved more effective than other methods of treating asthma. They are also considerably more expensive. Commercially available products are pressured and aerosolized much like a deodorant, and are often conveniently pocket-sized. Because they can be carried inconspicuously, some patients tend to overuse them.

Bronchodilators Administered Subcutaneously

Epinephrine hydrochloride (Adrenalin) and terbutaline sulfate (administered by injection) are often used in emergency rooms, but they have little value in the prolonged treatment of asthma patients. A patient overusing medications is an indication that the patient's medication program must be changed. The side effects of such medications are similar to those mentioned for other bronchodilators; they should be used cautiously in adults with cardiac problems or overactive thyroid glands.

Nontheophylline Bronchodilators Given Orally

In addition to theophylline discussed above, metaproterenol and terbutaline (Bricanyl and Brethine) are described as "more specific" in the marketing literature; that is, they cause bronchial smooth muscle dilation, or relaxation, without having an appreciable effect on the heart. Ephedrine, a component of such combination products as Tedral, can be useful in treating some individuals when it is given around the clock in conjunction with theophylline drugs. All the above-mentioned oral agents should be used with caution in patients suffering from high blood pressure, heart disease, hyperthyroidism, or respiratory failure.

Cromolyn Sodium

Cromolyn sodium (disodium cromoglycate), also called Intal, is a powder that can be propelled into the lungs by a special device called a spinhaler. Unlike the medications discussed above, which produce an immediate bronchodilatory response, cromolyn is a preventive medication. Patients will not benefit immediately, and, because of cromolyn sodium's occasional irritant qualities, some may develop slight bronchoconstriction. The irritation can be lessened and the penetration improved by using cromolyn after an aerosolized bronchodilator. Occasionally, a trial period of four to six weeks is indicated before the patient can be categorized as a nonresponder.

Oral Corticosteroids

When maximally tolerated doses of the medications discussed above are inadequate to control symptoms, corticosteroids might be used. As with any other medication, though, one must weigh the beneficial effects against possible side effects, and both benefits and side effects should be explained to the patient. Weight gain is a side effect that is often overlooked. Other side effects are given in Table 9.1. Although all the effects listed are possible adverse ones, they are also related to the duration of treatment, the dosage, and the timing of steroid therapy, as well as to the type of preparation given. Patients fear—sometimes irrationally—corticosteroids more than any other asthma medication. This medication can be lifesaving if carefully administered. By giving corticosteroids every other morning, and in small doses, the side effects can be almost totally eliminated. Long-acting preparations such as triamcinolone acetonide and dexamethasone, and sustained-action intramuscular preparations, are not given in an alternative-day program. By contrast, short-acting preparations such as prednisone, prednisolone, and methylprednisolone (Medrol) are preferable to long-acting preparations and are ideal alternate-day corticosteroid regimens. If a physician wishes to change the daily dosage schedule to an alternate-day schedule, three to four times the normal daily dose may initially be required. During an upper respiratory infection or other stress, a larger amount of prednisone or methylprednisolone can be administered for a few days; then the previous alternate-day schedule should be resumed. With such a short-term boost, side effects are minimal and temporary, and the alternate-day program can be reinstated immediately. If a patient has taken corticosteroids during the past year or has been on maintenance doses, corticosteroid supplements such as those mentioned above should be given during periods of stress—for example, during surgery. ACTH, a hormone secreted by the pituitary gland to stimulate the body to secrete its own steroids from the adrenal glands, has not proved an advantage over corticosteroids. Although commonly used in Europe, ACTH has certain disadvantages that make its use in the United States undesirable.

Table 9.1. Side Effects Associated with the Excessive Use of Corticosteroids

---

Cataracts
High blood pressure
Increased appetite
Low body potassium
Menstrual irregularities (women)
Muscle weakness
Peptic ulcer, gastric hypersecretion, or esophagitis
Psychological disturbances
Skin and body changes, such as acne, striae and skin bruises, and obesity
Growth suppression
Swelling of the body
Thinning of the bones
Unmasking or aggravating diabetes mellitus

Aerosolized Corticosteroids

Beclomethasone dipropionate (Vanceril), a recently marketed aerosolized corticosteroid, has proved effective in treating some patients. Although the drug has benefited many patients its effect has been most dramatic among those who require large daily doses of steroids. Beclomethasone is strongly advised for patients who are not doing well on more than four pills of prednisone (or an equivalent) on an alternate-day schedule. The prednisone should not be discontinued too rapidly while a patient is being switched from oral steroids to aerosolized steroids, or adrenal insufficiency could result. As mentioned in the discussion of cromolyn sodium, these medications are used as a means of prevention; they will not help during an acute attack. Occasionally, the medication may have to be discontinued if the Freon propellants aggravate the asthma symptoms. Once the aerosolized corticosteroids are broken down in the body the end products are not particularly active. Their effect, then, is a local one, much like the effect of steroid cream on a rash. Patients should be cautioned against overusing this medication, because it will also suppress the pituitary adrenal axis and may cause more general steroid side effects. The most common side effect is thrush, an easily treated fungus infection in the mouth that produces white patches discernible on the tongue and in the throat. There is probably an increased risk of developing thrush when antibiotics and large doses of oral corticosteroids are used together with an aerosol. Other contributing causes are diabetes and poor dental hygiene. The patient should be instructed to rinse the mouth after each treatment, either with an alcohol-based solution or with water. If these measures are not effective, the physician may have to prescribe a specific antifungal mouthwash.

Antibiotics

Antibiotics may be effective in treating some patients, while in others they may have no effect. In general, antibiotic therapy should be reserved for asthmatic patients with bacterial infections believed to contribute to bronchial obstruction. Antibiotics frequently are given empirically and before recurring data which report the identity of the organism that caused the infection. Asthmatics and bronchitics who chronically produce sputum may benefit from antibiotic therapy even though no specific causative bacteria have been identified. In such cases, broad-action spectrum antibiotics such as ampicillin or tetracycline can be prescribed along with a therapy that promotes good bronchial hygiene. Under these circumstances, antibiotics sometimes work because they decrease the total number of bacteria.

Mucolytics and Expectorants

The administration of fluids is the best way to thin secretions. Sometimes the fluids are given intravenously. Some fluids may be given with a nebulizer which, when combined with postural drainage and aerosolized bronchodilators, can be useful. Expectorants such as a saturated solution of potassium iodide (SSKI) or guanefesin have limited usefulness.

Less Commonly Used Medications

Atropine sulfate has been used as an aerosol and is helpful to some patients. Antihistamines also may provide relief of asthma in certain patients, but, because of their drying properties, they should be discontinued if it becomes difficult for the patient to bring up sputum. Other medications—for example, the antibiotic troleandomycin and such alpha adrenergic blocking agents as phentolamine—have specific but limited uses and should be given only under the supervision of a physician.

Tranquilizers and Sedatives

As is true of any drug, tranquilizers should be administered cautiously. Sometimes tranquilizers are administered to asthmatic patients in an attempt to counteract the stimulant effect of a bronchodilator. Because an anxious patient may also manifest a low level of oxygen in the blood, tranquilizers or sedatives should never be used when this condition is suspected. Instead, treatment with oxygen is usually recommended.

Allergy Injections

Allergy shots, also called immunotherapy or hyposensitization, are advised for certain cases when allergens such as pollens or molds are believed to contribute to the asthma, and when the elimination of these allergens from the environment is not practical. The group in which immunotherapy may prove most effective will, it is hoped, be better defined with improved diagnostic techniques such as bronchial inhalation challenges. Better control of studies is needed in evaluating immunotherapy for treating asthma patients.

Although asthma is a chronic disease characterized by periodic bronchial obstruction, patients who understand their illnesses and medication programs, and who are willing to work closely with their physicians, can expect to live a relatively normal, productive life.

Allergy Centers and Clinics

Major Allergy Centers and Clinics

The following is a list of the major allergy centers and clinics at hospitals around the country. The clinics offer care for allergy sufferers on an outpatient basis. Although this list is not intended to be comprehensive, it is a useful reference source in finding an allergy center or clinic in your area. The local chapters of the Asthma & Allergy Foundation of America, as well as the other associations listed in Appendix C, may be of help in locating an allergy clinic near you.

Note: The hospitals are listed in alphabetical order by state and then by city.

Arkansas

University of Arkansas Medical
  Center
4301 W. Markham St.
Little Rock, AR 72201
(501) 661-5000

California

Los Angeles–USC Medical Center
1200 N. State St.
Los Angeles, CA 90033
(213) 226-6503

UCLA Hospital
10833 Le Conte Ave.
Los Angeles, CA 90024
(213) 825-6481

University of California–Irvine
  Medical Center
101 City Dr., South
Orange, CA 92668
(714) 634-6011

Children's Hospital at Stanford
520 Willow Rd.
Palo Alto, CA 94304
(415) 327-4800

Kaiser Foundation Hospital
2200 O'Farrell
San Francisco, CA 94115
(415) 929-4000

University of California Hospitals
  and Clinics
513 Parnassus Ave.
San Francisco, CA 94143
(415) 666-9000

Stanford University Medical Center
300 Pasteur Dr.
Stanford, CA 94305
(415) 497-2300

Harbor General Hospital
1000 West Carson St.
Torrance, CA 90509
(213) 533-2104

Colorado

Fitzsimons Army Medical Center
Peoria and Colfax Sts.
Denver, CO 80240
(303) 341-8281

National Asthma Center
1999 Julian St.
Denver, CO 80204
(303) 458-1999

National Jewish Hospital
3800 E. Colfax Ave.
Denver, CO 80206
(303) 388-4461

University of Colorado Medical
   Center
4200 E. Ninth Ave.
Denver, CO 80262
(303) 394-7601

Connecticut

Yale–New Haven Medical Center
333 Cedar St.
New Haven, CT 06510
(203) 436-8060

District of Columbia

Children's Hospital National
   Medical Center
111 Michigan Ave.
Washington, DC 20010
(202) 745-5000

Georgetown University Hospital
3800 Reservoir Rd. NW
Washington, DC 20007
(202) 625-7001

Howard University Hospital
2041 Georgia Ave. NW
Washington, DC 20060
(202) 745-1596

Florida

William A. Shands Teaching
   Hospital and Clinics
University of Florida
Gainesville, FL 32610
(904) 392-3771

Illinois

Institute of Allergy & Clinical
   Immunology
Grant Hospital of Chicago
550 West Webster Ave.
Chicago, IL 60614
(312) 883-2000

Michael Reese Hospital and
   Medical Center
508 East 29th St.
Chicago, IL 60616
(312) 791-2000

Northwestern University Memorial
   Hospital
Superior St. and Fairbanks Ct.
Chicago, IL 60611
(312) 649-8624

Rush–Presbyterian–St. Luke's
   Medical Center
1753 W. Congress Pkwy.
Chicago, IL 60612
(312) 942-5000

University of Illinois Hospital
1919 W. Taylor St.
Chicago, IL 60612
(312) 996-7000

Kansas

University of Kansas College of
   Health Sciences and Bell
   Memorial Hospital
39th St. and Rainbow Blvd.
Kansas City, KS 66103
(913) 588-6008

Maryland

Good Samaritan Hospital
5601 Loch Raven Blvd.
Baltimore, MD 21239
(301) 323-2200

Johns Hopkins Hospital
601 N. Broadway
Baltimore, MD 21205
(301) 955-5000

Massachusetts

Massachusetts General Hospital
Clinical Immunology & Allergy
Unit
Fruit St.
Boston, MA 02114
(617) 726-2000

Robert B. Brigham Hospital
125 Parker Hill Ave.
Boston, MA 02120
(617) 732-5055

Michigan

University Hospital
1405 E. Ann St.
Ann Arbor, MI 48109
(313) 764-3184

Henry Ford Hospital
2799 West Grand Blvd.
Detroit, MI 48202
(313) 876-2600

Minnesota

University of Minnesota Hospitals
and Clinics
516 Delaware St.
Minneapolis, MN 55455
(612) 373-8484

Mayo Clinic and Foundation
200 First St. SW
Rochester, MN 55901
(507) 284-2511

Missouri

Children's Mercy Hospital
24th St. and Gillham Rd.
Kansas City, MO 64108
(816) 234-3000

Barnes Hospital–Washington
University Medical School
Barnes Hospital Plaza
St. Louis, MO 63110
(314) 454-2000

St. Louis University Medical Center
1402 S. Grand Blvd.
St. Louis, MO 63104
(314) 664-9800

Nebraska

St. Joseph Hospital
(formerly Creighton Hospital)
601 N. 30th St.
Omaha, NB 68131
(402) 449-4001

New York

Jewish Hospital and Medical Center
of Brooklyn
555 Prospect Pl.
Brooklyn, NY 11238
(212) 240-1761

Children's Hospital of Buffalo
219 Bryant St.
Buffalo, NY 14222
(716) 878-7000

Nassau County Medical Center
2201 Hempstead Tpk.
East Meadow, NY 11554
(516) 542-0123

R. A. Cooke Institute of Allergy—
Roosevelt Hospital
428 West 59th St.
New York, NY 10028
(212) 554-7000

Cornell Medical School—
New York Hospital
510 East 70th St.
New York, NY 10021
(212) 472-5900

New York University Medical
Center
552 First Ave.
New York, NY 10016
(212) 340-5241

Ohio

Children's Hospital Medical Center
Elland and Bethesda Aves.
Cincinnati, OH 45229
(513) 559-4200

Cleveland Clinic Foundation
9500 Euclid Ave.
Cleveland, OH 44106
(216) 444-5780

Ohio State University Hospitals
456 Clinic Dr.
Columbus, OH 43210
(614) 422-4851

Pennsylvania

Children's Hospital of Philadelphia
34th St. and Civic Center Blvd.
Philadelphia, PA 19104
(215) 596-9100

Hahnemann Medical College and
Hospital
Feinstein Bldg.
216 North Broad St.
Philadelphia, PA 19102
(215) 448-7000

Hospital of University of
Pennsylvania
34th and Spruce Sts.
Philadelphia, PA 19104
(215) 662-4000

Thomas Jefferson University
Hospital
11th and Walnut Sts.
Philadelphia, PA 19107
(215) 928-6000

Children's Hospital of Pittsburgh
125 De Soto St.
Pittsburgh, PA 15213
(412) 647-2345

Rhode Island

Rhode Island Hospital
593 Eddy St.
Providence, RI 02902
(401) 277-4000

Texas

University of Texas Health Sciences
Center
7703 Floyd Curl Dr.
San Antonio, TX 78284
(512) 691-6011

University of Texas Medical
Branch Hospitals
8th and Mechanic Sts.
Galveston, TX 77550
(713) 765-1011

Texas Children's Hospital—Baylor
College of Medicine
6621 Fannin
Houston, TX 77030
(713) 791-4219

Virginia

University of Virginia Hospitals
Private Clinic Bldg.
Hospital Dr.
Charlottesville, VA 22908
(804) 924-0211

Medical College of Virginia
Hospitals
12th and Marshall Sts.
Richmond, VA 23298
(804) 786-9000

Washington

University Hospital
1959 NE Pacific St.
Seattle, WA 98195
(206) 543-3300

Wisconsin

University of Wisconsin Hospital
and Clinics
600 Highland Ave.
Madison, WI 53702
(608) 263-8000

The following institutions comprise a national network for scientific and clinical studies in asthma and allergic diseases and are supported by the Federal government's focus of research in immunology, the National Institute of Allergy and Infectious Diseases.

Centers for Interdisciplinary Research on Immunologic Diseases

California

UCLA School of Medicine
Center for Health Sciences Building
Los Angeles, CA 90024

District of Columbia

Georgetown University School of
Medicine
3900 Reservoir Road, N.W.
Washington, DC 20007

Maryland

The Johns Hopkins University
School of Medicine
Good Samaritan Hospital
5601 Loch Raven Boulevard
Baltimore, MD 21239

Massachusetts

Children's Hospital Medical Center
300 Longwood Avenue
Boston, MA 02115

Missouri

Washington University School of
Medicine
660 South Euclid Avenue
St. Louis, MO 63110

New York

University of Rochester
School of Medicine and Dentistry
601 Elmwood Avenue
Rochester, NY 14642

Asthma and Allergic Diseases Centers

California
Scripps Clinic and Research
Foundation
10666 North Torrey Pines Road
La Jolla, CA 92037

UCSD Medical Center
225 Dickinson Center
San Diego, CA 92103

University of California at
  San Francisco
Department of Medicine
400 Parnassus Avenue
San Francisco, CA 94143

Illinois

Northwestern University Medical
  School
303 East Chicago Avenue
Chicago, IL 60611

Iowa

University of Iowa Hospitals
Department of Internal Medicine
Division of Allergy & Immunology
Iowa City, IA 52242

Louisiana

Tufts University School of
  Medicine
1700 Perdido Street
New Orleans, LA 70112

Tulane University School of
  Medicine
1700 Perdido Street
New Orleans, LA 70112

Maryland

National Institutes of Health,
  NIAID
Building 10, Room 11N250
Bethesda, MD 20205

Massachusetts

Harvard Medical School
75 Francis Street
Boston, MA 02115

New York

The Rockefeller University
1230 York Avenue
New York, NY 10021

State University of New York at
  Stony Brook
Health Sciences Center
Stony Brook, NY 11794

North Carolina

Duke University
Box 2898
Durham, NC 27710

Texas

University of Texas Health Science
  Center
Dermatology Division
5223 Harry Hiyes Boulevard
Dallas, TX 75235

Wisconsin

Medical College of Wisconsin
Department of Medicine
8700 West Wisconsin Avenue
Box 12
Milwaukee, WI 53226

Summer Camps for Allergic and Asthmatic Children

A number of summer camps across the United States specialize in the care of children with health problems and have developed special programs to meet their needs. Some camps admit children with all kinds of health problems; others are organized only for allergic and asthmatic children. Some parents may feel that their child's asthma or allergy isn't severe enough to warrant sending the child to a special camp. For parents who do not choose a summer camp that specializes in asthmatic and allergic children, The Asthma & Allergy Foundation of America suggests the following criteria:

Are animals likely to be found near living quarters?
Is a doctor available on a full-time basis?
Will medicine and injections be given when needed?
Does the camp have alternatives to sports, such as an arts and crafts program?

Following is a list of camps, by state, with facilities and/or programs designed for allergic and asthmatic children. Camps preceded by an asterisk (*) are accredited by the American Camping Association.

Arizona

Friendly Pines Camp
Senator Rd.
Prescott, AZ 86301
(602) 252-2128
  Contact: Mr. or Mrs. May, owners
  Facilities and activities: 160-acre, pollen-free, Western riding camp in the Ponderosa Pine Forest.

Medical care: A fully equipped infirmary with a full-time registered nurse.
  Comment: The camp is not organized specifically for asthmatics, although some asthmatic children do attend it for the beneficial climate.
  Fee: $800 for the first four-week session; $835 for the second four-week session.

Arkansas

*Alders Gate
2000 Alders Gate Rd.
Little Rock, AK 72205
(501) 225-1444
Contact: Bruce Tomasson, camp coordinator
Facilities and activities: Lake for swimming and fishing in a rural setting and 2 therapeutic pools. Counselors and volunteers supervise activities. The camp is barrier-free for the physically handicapped.
Medical care: The camp has a medical staff with a full-time registered nurse and, for emergencies, access to a nearby medical center.
Comment: One week during each summer is dedicated to children with lung-related problems.
Fee: $200 per camper/week with limited funds available for scholarship.

California

*Boys Club Camp #365
Running Springs, CA 92382
Contact: Lorraine Nelson, Secretary-Treasurer
Asthma & Allergy Foundation of America
Los Angeles Chapter
(213) 326-5357
Camp Director: Dr. Roger Katz
(213) 645-1616
Facilities and activities: The camp is pollution- and pollen-free, with group cabins that have no feather bedding. Typical regular activities are riflery, archery, and swimming in a heated pool. Ice skating and fishing trips are conducted outside the camp. Animals are kept away from the immediate vicinity.
Medical care: One full-time registered nurse, six doctors on call, and an infirmary.

Comment: The camp's program is tailored to the needs of moderate and severe asthmatics.
Fee: No fee for the 10 day session.

*Hollywood Camp
3200 Canyon Dr.
Los Angeles, CA 90068
(213) 467-7193
Director: Joe McElvogne
Facilities and activities: Campers are housed in cabins and are mainstreamed with other campers. The camp offers backpacking, archery, music, drama, dancing, horseback riding, hiking, environmental education, crafts, rowing, canoeing, and aquatics.
Fees: Girls from 7 to 14, coed 7 to 14, adults; 5 days for $65.00, 2 days for $24.00, 3 days for $32.00. Operating season 1/1 to 12/31.

*Sequoia Lake Family
Sequoia Lake
Miramonte, CA 93654
(209) 335-2886
Director: Larry Lower
(209) 233-7788
Facilities and activities: A-frame cabins also with cabins, dorms, tents and a lodge. The camp offers softball, football, basketball, archery, drama, dance, hiking, environmental education, crafts, sailing, and aquatics.
Fees: Coed from 10 to 18, adults from 18 to 99; 4 days for $84.00, 7 days from $140.00 to $795.00, depending on programs chosen.

Connecticut

*Lenox Hill Camp
North Shore Rd.
Bantam, CT 067500400
(203) 567-9760

Director: Walter Thompson
(212) 744-5022

Facilities and activities: Cabins and a lodge. The camp offers field sports, archery, outdoor living skills, environmental education, crafts, rowing, and aquatics.

Fees: Coed from 7 to 15, from 60+; 20 days for $350.00.

*Camp Shalom
425 Meriman Rd.
Windsor, CT 06095
(203) 688-4202

Director: David L. Jacobs
(203) 236-4571

Facilities and activities: Campers are housed in cabins. The camp offers field sports, tennis, archery, music, outdoor living skills, mountaineering, horseback riding, environmental education, crafts, sailing, and aquatics.

Fees: Coed from 5 to 15; 10 days for $190.00, 20 days for $390.00, 30 days for $577.00, 40 days for $796.00.

Idaho

*Camp Easter Seal East
Worley, ID 83876

Contact: Diane Albright,
Camp Director
Easter Seal Camp Program
521 Second Ave., West
Seattle, WA 98119
(206) 284-5706

Facilities and activities: The camp —located on forty acres, which includes a lakefront—provides the standard camp activities of arts and crafts, as well as water and other sports, drama, and music. Horses are excluded.

Medical care: The camp has an infirmary with an isolation ward, an examination room, and six beds. It is staffed by a minimum of two full-time nurses, with a physician on call. A standing arrangement for emergencies has been made with a local hospital and the Fairchild Air Force Base.

Comment: The only requirement of the camp is that a child be able to use the camp's recreational facilities.

Fee: $74 to $100 for a one-week session. There are two sessions each summer, divided by age group. An arrangement called a campership is available for those unable to pay the full fee.

Illinois

*Camp AAFA at Camp
Ravenswood
20950 West Grand Ave.
P.O. Box 306
Lake Villa, IL 60046

Contact: Pat Koutouzos
(312) 747-9533

Applications and information:
(312) 755-0750

Facilities and activities: Camp AAFA is conducted at the facility of Camp Ravenswood. Activities included are swimming, canoeing, many ball sports, hiking, and arts and crafts.

Medical care: The camp is staffed by a doctor, nurse, and a registered allergist as well as YMCA staff counselors.

Comment: All allergy and asthma victims attending are mainstreamed with the other campers attending.

Fee: $150.00 for the 4- to 6-day session. Camperships are available to those in need of financial assistance.

Algonquin
Cary Rd.
Algonquin, IL 60102
(312) 658-8212

Director: Jane T. Pirsug
(312) 461-0800

Facilities and activities: Campers are housed in cabins, dorms, and tents. The camp offers softball, snow activities, outdoor living skills, hiking, farming, environmental education, sailing, rowing, and aquatics.

Fee: Coed from 1 to 12, adults from 20 to 60, adults from 60 to 95, payments based on a sliding scale.

Indiana

*Julia Jameson Health Camp for Children, Inc.
Office: 1100 West 42nd Street
Indianapolis, IN 46208
(317) 923-3925
Camp: 201 South Bridgeport Rd.
Indianapolis, IN 46231

Contact: Ed Nelson, director

Facilities and activities: One large building, which includes sleeping quarters; a small infirmary, with two isolation rooms and a medical dispensary that is available at all times; a barn for activities; and a small, shallow pool for swimming.

Medical care: During regular sessions, a staff nurse is on duty and three pediatricians are on call. During special sessions, three nurses, three respiratory therapists, and a medical doctor are available.

Comment: Children with general health problems, including asthmatics without serious conditions, are accepted during the camp's regular three-week sessions. At midsummer, the American Lung Association of Central Indiana sponsors special one-week sessions for asthmatic children. The sessions are restricted to residents of eight counties in the standard Indianapolis metropolitan area.

Fee: $200 for a three-week session, but the fee is based on ability to pay; all children are accepted regardless of the ability to pay. One-week sessions for asthmatics are conducted, which cost $100; scholarships are available from the American Lung Association of Central Indiana.

Kentucky

*Camp Green Shores
Star Route One, Box 261
McDaniels, KY 40152
(502) 257-2508

Contact: Camping and Recreation Department, Kentucky Easter Seal Society.

Camp director: Jim Watkins

Facilities and activities: A five-room health-care facility that includes an isolation room, cabins, a lakefront with boating equipment, an outdoor swimming pool, an arts-and-crafts program, outdoor camping and cooking, and horseback riding.

Medical care: Access to a local hospital; two full-time nurses, one of whom is a registered nurse; and local doctors on call.

Comment: The camp caters to children with medical problems that prevent them from attending regular camps.

Fee: $400 for an 11-day session, with four sessions each summer. Payment is according to ability to pay, based on a sliding scale.

*Camp Kysoc
1902 Easterday Rd.
Carrollton, KY 41008
(502) 732-5333

Contact: Camping and Recreation Department, Kentucky Easter Seal Society.

Camp director: Sally Bunnell

Facilities and activities: A five-room health-care facility, including an isolation room; cabins; lakefront and boating equipment; an outdoor swimming pool; arts and crafts, and outdoor camping and cooking.

Medical care: Two full-time nurses, one of whom is a registered nurse; local doctors on call; and access to a local hospital.

Comment: Geared to children with medical problems that prevent them from attending regular camps.

Fee: $380 for an eleven-day session, with five sessions each summer. Payment is according to ability to pay, based on a sliding scale.

Maryland

*Chesapeake Camp Centers
50 Happy Valley Rd.
Port Deposit, MD 21904
(301) 378-2261
Director: Lloyd Elling (301) 378-2261
Facilities and activities: Campers are housed in cabins, dorms, Logans, tents, teepees, and a lodge. The camp offers religion, music, drama, dance, outdoor living skills, leader training, horseback riding, hiking, crafts, canoeing, and aquatics.
Fees: Boys from 8 to 15, girls from 8 to 15; 7 days for $185.00, 14 days for $355.00, 21 days for $510.00, 28 days for $660.00.

Massachusetts

*Caraban Society for Children
P. O. Box 357
Athol, MA 01331
(617) 249-6010
Director: Donald Castine (617) 249-4845

Facilities and activities: Campers are housed in cabins and dorms. The camp offers crafts, arts, and aquatics.
Fees: Coed from 5 to 15; 7 days for $100.00.

*Northeastern
The Warren Center
529 Chestnut St.
Ashland, MA 01721
(617) 881-1142
Director: Paul Mentag (617) 881-4142
Facilities and activities: Campers reside in cabins, tents, and a lodge. The camp offers backpacking, canoe tripping, team field sports, tennis, archery, outdoor living skills, leader training, hiking, crafts, sailing, canoeing, and swimming instruction.
Fees: Coed from 8 to 14; 12 days for $260.00.

Minnesota

*Mischawake
Box 368
Grand Rapids, MN 55744
(218) 326-5011
Director: Norman Ericson
Facilities and activities: Campers reside in cabins, tents, or a lodge. The camp offers camping, team sports, tennis, riflery, archery, music, drama, outdoor living skills, leader training, horseback riding, hiking, crafts, sailing, and aquatics.
Fees: Boys from 8 to 16, girls from 8 to 16, adults from 20 to 99; 28 days for $950.00, 56 days from $1850.00.

*Superkids
1829 Portland Ave.
Minneapolis, MN 55404
(612) 871-7332

Contact: Cathy Hall, camp co-ordinator

Director: Penny Gottier (612) 872-7332

Facilities and activities: Campers reside in cabins. The camp offers trip camping, team sports, riflery, archery, individual sports, music, drama, outdoor living skills, leader training, horseback riding, crafts, sailing, rowing, and aquatics.

Medical care: An infirmary staffed by three full-time physicians, ten nurses, and two pharmacists, all available on a twenty-four-hour basis.

Comment: The camp—sponsored by the American Lung Association of Hennepin County, the Minnesota Lung Association—is located on the shore of Lake Independence, just outside Minneapolis.

Fees: Coed from 7 to 14; 6 days for $110.00; 12 days from $215.00.

Missouri

*Day Camp Safari
9116 Lackland Rd.
St. Louis, MO 63114
(314) 428-0840

Director: Tom Ersland

Facilities and activities: Camp is day only. The camp offers field sports, gymnastics, archery, outdoor living skills, crafts, art, and aquatics.

Fees: Coed from 5 to 13; 10 days for $55.50, 5 days for $42.50.

New Jersey

*Vacamas, Inc.
256 Macopin Rd.
West Milford, NJ 07480
(201) 492-0204

Director: Michael Friedman (201) 492-0204

Facilities and activities: Campers are housed in cabins and tents. The camp offers canoe tripping, back-packing, field sports, outdoor living skills, leader training, hiking, rowing, canoeing, arts, and aquatics.

Fees: Coed from 8 to 16. Fees are on a sliding scale based on the ability to pay.

New York

*Hidden Valley Camp
Sharpe Reservation
Route 3
Fishkill, NY 12524
(914) 897-9860

Contact: Pamela Galehouse, Fresh Air Fund (212) 586-0200

Facilities and activities: An air-conditioned infirmary, a heated pool, two lakes on twenty-five hundred acres, winterized cabins, a planetarium, and a model farm. Partially barrier-free.

Medical care: Two full-time registered nurses, four pediatricians on call within a three-mile radius.

Comment: The camp, for residents of New York City only, is owned and operated by the Fresh Air Fund. It is nonprofit, financed by private contributions.

Fee: No fee; for low-income families only.

*Wagon Road Camp
Chappaqua, NY 10514

Contact: Richard Steinberg, Director (914) 238-8106

Facilities and activities: A clinic, six-bed infirmary, and separate housing on fifty-two acres. Children suffering from similar problems share cabins; there is roughly one staff member for every two campers. The camp has a well-rounded program, consisting of crafts, athletics, music and drama, nature study, and swimming in a heated pool. All programs except swimming are open to both ambulatory and nonambulatory children.

Medical care: Two pediatricians on call at all times, and two full-time registered nurses. The services of a consulting allergist are also available.

Comment: The camp has been owned and operated by the Children's Aid Society since 1955. It is inspected by the state.

Fee: $400 for 3 weeks but is based on the ability to pay.

*Frost Valley YMCA Camps
Olivera, NY 12462
(914) 985-7400
Director: Michael Ketcham (201) 838-4495
Facilities and activities: Campers stay in cabins, tents, teepees, or the lodge. The camp offers trip camping, field sports, gymnastics, archery, ranching, physical fitness, performing arts, outdoor living skills, hiking, cycling, sailing, and aquatics.
Fees: Boys and girls from 7 to 16, adults from 18 to 99; 17 days for $325.00, 6 days for $165.00.

Ohio

*Camp Allyn
Amelia Olive Branch Rd.
Batavia, OH 45103
(513) 732-0240
Contact: Irene Taylor, Director.
Facilities and activities: Heated pool, sleeping units, dining hall, covered pavillion game room;

hospital nearby; arts and crafts, boating, swimming, and nature studies.

Medical care: A full-time registered nurse and, during the special season for asthmatics, a full-time doctor.

Comment: This camp grew out of a pilot program begun in 1980 for asthmatic children aged 8 to 13. The camp is operated by the southwestern Ohio Lung Association. Oher camp programs are open to people aged 6 to 65 with many, varied handicaps. There are four twelve-day sessions and special six-day program especially designed for asthmatics.

Fee: For the twelve-day session, the fee is left up to parents, based on their ability to pay; for the six-day session, there is a small fee.

*Evergreen
4646 Pampel Rd.
Houston, OH 453339797
(513) 492-0785
Director: Michael Hanback (513) 323-3781
Facilities and activities: Campers are housed in the lodge, cabins, or tents. The camp offers soccer, team sports, archery, fitness, band, mountaineering, horseback riding, hiking, environmental education, crafts, rowing, canoeing, and aquatics.
Fees: Coed from 6 to 18, adults from 18 to 65; 6 days for $85.00, 3 days for $45.00, and 6 days for $65.00.

*Stepping Stones
5650 Given Rd.
Cincinnati, OH 45243
(513) 831-4660
Contact: Lucy Smith, Director
Facilities and activities: Twenty-three acres, with twelve-unit sites

to which campers are assigned according to age, ability, and interest; indoor and outdoor heated pools, arts and crafts, boating, and nature studies. A hospital is nearby.

Medical care: A full-time registered nurse.

Comment: This is a day camp only. People with any handicap are accepted, with age groups ranging from infants to the elderly.

Fee: $15.60 per day.

Virginia

*Holiday Trails
Route 1, Box 356
Charlottesville, VA 22901
(804) 977-3781

Contact: Ann Williams, Administrative Assistant

Facilities and activities: The camp is located on 72 pollen-free acres in the mountains, with a pool, lake, and infirmary. The usual camp activities—including arts and crafts, horseback riding, and sports —are provided.

Medical care: A full-time physician and two full-time, registered nurses.

Comment: Operated by a private, nonprofit organization, the camp is open to children with most types of medical problems except the mentally retarded and those who are confined to wheelchairs.

Fee: $350 for a two-week session, with one session each summer; $500 for a three-week session (two each summer). Camperships are available, and campers are accepted on a first-come-first-serve basis. No children are rejected because of inability to pay.

Washington

*Camp Easter Seals West
Contact: Paul Sorenson
17719 South Vaugh Rd.
Vaugh, Washington 98394
(206) 884-2722

Facilities and activities: The camp is located near a salt-water bay and offers horseback riding, camping, arts and crafts, and aquatics.

Medical care: The camp is staffed with a nurse, and a doctor is on call.

Comment: The camp meets the approval of the Easter Seals standards and is ACA affiliated.

Fee: $100.00 per week. $65.00 for 4-day session.

Wisconsin

*Easter Seal Center for Camping
& Recreation
Contact: Ken Saville, Director of Camping and Recreation
Camp Wawbeek Pioneer Camp
Wisconsin Dells, WI 53965
(608) 254-8319 (summer);
(608) 231-3411 (year-round)

Facilities and activities: Campers are housed in cabins, dorms, tents, and the lodge. The camp offers hockey, baseball, music, drama, band, horseback riding, environmental education, cycling, crafts, rowing and canoeing, and aquatics.

Fees: Coed from 8 to 17, adults from 18 to 60; 12 days for $400.00. Scholarships are available to Wisconsin residents.

Canada

*Illahee Northwoods Camp
22 Wellesley St.

Toronto, Ontario M4Y 1G3
Canada
(416) 922-3126
Contact: Director
Facilities and activities: The
camp is located on 140 acres of
woods, fields, and game areas and
provides swimming, sailing, canoeing, crafts, and hiking in a pollen-
free environment. It has an infirmary, and a hospital is nearby for
emergencies.
Medical care: One doctor and
two nurses in residence at all times.
A qualified dietician plans meals.

Comment: Programs are carefully supervised to meet the needs
of children with health problems,
including those with asthma and
allergies.
Fee: For residents of metropolitan Toronto, fees are based on
ability to pay; for those outside
metropolitan Toronto the fee is
$495 for 2 weeks, $990 for 4
weeks.

* Denotes approved American
Camping Association Camp.

Allergy Associations

Chapters of The Allergy & Asthma Foundation of America

The Asthma & Allergy Foundation of America
1302 18th Street NW Suite 303
Washington, D.C. 20036
(202) 293-2950

The national headquarters office of The Asthma & Allergy Foundation of America provides staff support for this important, fast-growing voluntary health organization. It is a national resource for information about asthma and allergic diseases needed by professionals, patients, and the general public. It produces and disseminates valuable publications and other educational aids to groups and organizations, publishes the Asthma & Allergy ADVANCE (the nation's only regular newspaper devoted to the interests of the millions with asthma and allergic diseases), and coordinates a broad range of educational and fund-raising programs through local chapters, listed below.

Chapter and Support Groups

California

Los Angeles Chapter
Mickie Faris, MPH, Exec. Dir.
Suite 1005
5410 Wilshire Blvd.
Los Angeles, CA 90036
(213) 937-7859
    Sidney Levenson, MD
    President

San Diego & Imperial Counties
    Chapter
7920 Frost St., #100
San Diego, CA 92123
(619) 292-1144
    Judy Bachman, Ph.D.
    Acting President

Redwood Empire Chapter
P.O. Box 4688
Santa Rosa, CA 95401
(707) 527-7456
    Sheri Graves
    President

District of Columbia

Metropolitan Washington Chapter
P.O. Box 1631
Rockville, MD 20850
(301) 424-6617
    Eileen Rosenthal
    President

Florida

Florida Gulf Coast Chapter
708 Del Prado Blvd.
Cape Coral, FL 33904
(813) 574-0347
(813) 936-0344
  Ronald Wyatt
  President

South Florida Chapter
3181 NW 108th Dr.
Coral Springs, FL 33021
(305) 752-2917
  Jo Combs
  President

Illinois

Greater Chicago Chapter
111 North Wabash, Suite 909
Chicago, IL 60602
(312) 346-0745
  Virginia Osorio
  President

Louisiana

Louisiana Chapter
2507 Napoleon Ave.
New Orleans, LA 70115
(504) 899-4639
(504) 899-3527
  W. Wayne Lake, Jr., M.D.
  President

Maryland

Maryland Chapter
Beverly Caporossi, Exec. Sec.
5601 Loch Raven Blvd.
Baltimore, MD 21239
(301) 433-3950
  Phillip S. Norman, M.D.
  President

Massachusetts

New England Chapter
1 Walnut St.
Boston, MA 02108
(617) 742-7452
890 East St.
Tewksbury, MA 01876
  George D. Behrakis
  President

Missouri

St. Louis Chapter
P.O. Box 1664
Manchester, MO 63011
  Shirley O'Connor
  President

"Show Me" Chapter
Gail Tucker, Exec. Sec.
706 East Clark Ave.
Warrensburg, MO 64093
(816) 747-6930
  Maurine Achauer, Ph.D.
  President

New York

New York Chapter
20 East 9th St.
New York, NY 10003
(212) 741-4863 office
(212) 777-0505 home
  Laurie Bell
  President

Ohio

Miami Valley Chapter
1500 First National Bank Plaza
Dayton, OH 45402
(513) 222-4009
  Herman M. Lubens, M.D.
  President

Pennsylvania

Northeastern Pennsylvania Chapter
Box 28
Dalton, PA 18414
(717) 586-1404 office
  Richard Zepel, Ph.D.
  President

Southeastern Pennsylvania Chapter
P.O. Box 249
Plymouth Meeting, PA 19462
(215) 825-0582
  Edward K. Tryon
  President

Cumberland Valley Chapter
341 Strickler Ave.
Waynesboro, PA 17268
(717) 762-1880
  Janet Brockmann
  President

Tennessee

East Tennessee Chapter
P.O. Box 11289
Knoxville, TN 37923
  Alicia Hardin
  President

AAFA Pending Chapters

Minnesota

Minnesota Chapter
Box 434 Mayo
Department of Medicine,
Mayo Memorial Building
420 Delaware St., SE
Minneapolis, MN 55455
(612) 373-4330
  Malcolm N. Blumenthal, M.D.
  President

Ohio

Cincinnati Chapter.
2985 Spruceway Dr.
Cincinnati, OH 45247
(513) 851-3198
  Debra Teague
  President

Pennsylvania

Three Rivers Chapter
1119 8th Ave.
New Brighton, PA 15066
  Debbie Householder
  President

AAFA Support Groups

Noelle Albert
AAFA Support Group
7905 East 134th Terrace
Grandview, MO 64030

Fred Wheeler
AAFA Support Group
Route 1, Box 137
Winchester, VA 22601

Joseph J. Trautlein, M.D.
AAFA Support Group
Hershey Medical Center
Hershey, PA 17033

Other Allergy Associations

Following is a list of other allergy association in the United States and Canada, with a statement of purpose and the professional services offered for each association. For additional information on allergy treatment and allergy-related problems, the interested reader should write to specific associations. Note: The associations are given alphabetically, with U. S. and Canadian associations intermixed. Their primary orientation is listed as professional, patient and/or public.

Allergy Information Association
25 Poynter Dr., Room 7
Weston, Ontario M9R 1K8
Canada
(416) 244-9312
Patient and *Public*

American Academy of Allergy and
    Immunology
611 East Wells St.
Milwaukee, WI 53202
(414) 272-6071
Professional

American Allergy Association
P.O. Box 7273
Menlo Park, CA 94025
(415) 322-1663
Patient and *Public*

American Association of Certified
    Allergists
401 East Prospect Ave., Suite 210
Mount Prospect, IL 60056
(312) 255-1024
Professional

American Association for Clinical
    Immunology and Allergy
P.O. Box 912
Omaha, NE 68101
(402) 551-0801
Professional

American Board of Allergy and
    Immunology
    A conjoint board of the Amer-
ican Board of Internal Medicine
and the American Board of Pediatrics
3624 Science Center
Philadelphia, PA 19104
(215) 349-9466
Professional

American College of Allergists
2141 14th St.
Boulder, CO 80302
(303) 447-8111
Professional

American Society of
    Ophthalmologic and
    Otolaryngologic Allergy
Bowman Gray School of Medicine
Winston-Salem, NC 27103
(919) 727-4161
Professional

Association of Allergists for
    Mycological Investigations
444 Hermann Professional Building
610 Fannin St.
Houston, TX 77030
Professional

Histamine Club
Cornell University Medical College
1300 York Ave.
New York, NY 10021
(212) 472-5971
Professional

International Allergy Association
133 East 58th St.
New York, NY 10022
(212) 355-1005
Professional

International Correspondence
  Society of Allergists (ICSA)
139 South Grant Ave.
Columbus, OH 43215
(614) 221-2457
Professional

National Institute of Allergy
  and Infectious Diseases
9000 Rockville Pike
Bethesda, MD 20205
(301) 496-2263
Professional and *Public*

Index

Numbers in italics refer to illustrations

I

R

S

Salbutamol, 92
Salivary gland swelling, 9
Sauces, allergy-free, 194-95
Sauna taker's disease, 43
SCH-1000, 92
Scratch test, 56, 58
Seed allergens, 56, 147
Self-medication, 75
Sensitize, 56
Sequoiosis, 43
Serotonin, 56-57
Serum sickness, 32-33, 57, 113
Shellfish, 19, 68, 75, 186, 217
Shock organ, 57
Sinus disease, 2, 5, 9, 71, 73, 218-219
SK-Diphenhyramine, 86
Skin disease research, 130-31
Skin reactions, 70, 81-82
  emergency, 70
  See also Allergic dermatitis;
    Atopic dermatitis; Contact
    dermatitis; Eczema;
    Exfoliative dermatitis;
    Hives; Rashes; Urticaria
Skin tests, 10, 57-58, 116, 119,
  213
  for food allergies, 37, 164
Slow-reacting substance of
    anaphylaxis (SRS-A), 58
    119, 120
Smog, industrial, 14-15
Smoking, 4. *See also* Tobacco
  smoke
Solu-Medrol, 96
Soups, allergy-free, 189
Soybeans, 9, 37
Specificity, 58
Spin-Haler, 93, 223
Spirometer, 58

Spores, 58
Sputum, 58, 214
SSKI, 225
Status asthmaticus, 58
Stem cells, 103, 117
Steroids, *see* Corticosteroids;
    Cortisone
Stevens-Johnson syndrome, 33
Subcutaneous provocation
    testing, 139
Suberosis, 43
Sublingual provocation testing,
    139
Sudafed, 89
Sulfa drugs, 33
Surgical tape, 176
Swelling, 19
Symptoms (table), 67-68
Synthetic fabrics, 7-8
Systemic allergic reactions, 85
Systemic lupus erythematosus
    (SLE), 59

T

Tacaryl, 87
Tagamet, 87
Tartrazin, 218
Tavist, 86
T cells, 49, 59, 103-107, 121,
    129-130, 134, 136
  cytotoxic, 105, 130
  helper, 105, 115, 130
  suppressor, 105, 115, 122-23
  See also Lymphocytes
Tea allergy, 221
Tedral, 80, 221, 222
Temaril, 87
Terbutaline, 80, 91, 212, 222
Terbutaline sulfate, 216, 222
Tetrahydrozoline, 89
Thatched roof lung, 43